M000191932

Chana Klein

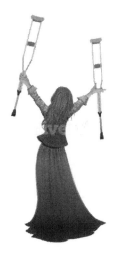

Mike,

May The Light of
Real Healing be yours
always
♡
Chana

Light FROM the Darkness
of Illness & Physical Disability

What Makes Us Ill
What Keeps Us Ill
& How to Heal

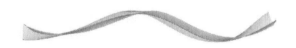

Chana Klein

Light FROM the Darkness
of Illness & Physical Disability

What Makes Us Ill
What Keeps Us Ill
& How to Heal
By Chana Klein

True Stories of Understanding
and Overcoming
Physical Illness & Disability

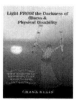

Copyright © 2018 Chana Klein

Light FROM the Darkness of Illness & Physical Disability

All rights reserved. No part of this book may be used or reproduced in any manner whatsoever without written permission except in the case of brief quotations embodied in critical articles or reviews using source info.

ISBN-13: 978-0692985779
ISBN-10: 0692985778

Cover illustration by Kokila Harshani
Cover Design by Prasanthika Mihiri
Both from Sri Lanka
Illustration Artists: Chana Klein, Rukmali
Fernando, & Kokila Harshani
Author Photograph by Heshie Klein, MD

Published by
Light FROM the Darkness Creations
New Jersey
2018

For information contact
chana@lightfromthedarkness.com

Chana Klein

CONTENTS

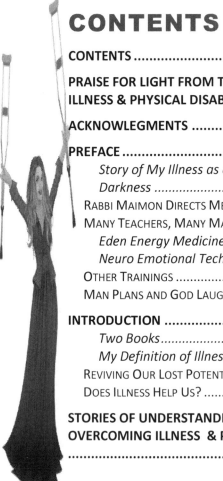

Chana Klein

PRAISE FOR LIGHT FROM THE DARKNESS OF ILLNESS & PHYSICAL DISABILITY

Chana Klein's **Light from the Darkness of Illness and Physical Disability** ranks among the best self-help books that one can read.

Based on sources, experts in their fields and empirical evidence, in this volume, Chana takes the reader through a host of health challenges that confront people.

Written in an engaging manner, the book argues persuasively that the human being can help himself/herself far more that is usually acknowledged.

Chana Klein's use of biblical personalities and Jewish thought in the self-help process is particularly interesting.

May Chana's approach help others just as it has sustained her through very dark times.

Chana Klein

The book radiates the warmth of light as it seeks to overcome the pain of darkness.

Rabbi Menahem Meier, Shlita

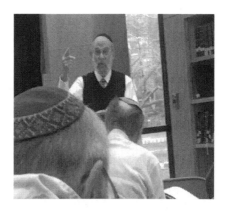

ACKNOWLEGMENTS

My first debt of gratitude is to The Almighty for the clarity and the excellent health He has granted me in writing this book.

Next, my deepest thanks to Rabbi Menahem Meier, Shlita, with whom I have been so fortunate to learn as one of his students for the past two years. I thank Rabbi Meier for reviewing my entire manuscript and for his invaluable suggestions, most of which were incorporated into the final draft.

I so appreciate his contribution.

I am grateful also, once again, to my ex-husband, Heshie Klein, MD, for taking an even better updated photo of me than the one he took last year, which turned out to be far superior to the one that a professional photographer had taken.

I thank him also, for his Herculean attention to every detail of spelling, Hebrew terms, grammar and phrasing in his reviewing every chapter as well as all the Internet links provided.

It is the rare person who is so busy with important things as are Rabbi Meier and Dr. Klein, yet will read a piece right away and give me feedback.

Those who do are precious to an author like me.

I thank also each of my teachers of Healing mentioned in this work as well as the many teachers of Torah with whom I learn every day.

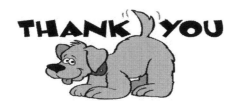

PREFACE

Years of illness, all kinds, from disability to inability, to deathly ill. That was me.

Incurable conditions, pain, feeling awful, physically, mentally, emotionally, and spiritually.

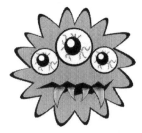

Light FROM the Darkness of Illness
& Physical Disability

Hopeless diagnoses with no known

remedies.

I have been there.

After a 34-year career as an educator, I was

led to working as a Mind-Body Practitioner,

a Healer, an ADHD/ASD/General Coach,

and a specialist in "Coaching the

Uncoachable", my favorite clients.

Chana Klein

Story of My Illness as a Light FROM the Darkness

I was a teacher.
I thrived on being a teacher.
I had no interest in, or intention of
becoming a healer.

I loved the classroom and was sure that
Heaven for me will be a classroom of kids,
for it has always been the faces of the
children with whom I worked that filled me
with endless energy and joy.

Light FROM the Darkness of Illness & Physical Disability

I planned on being a teacher for the rest of my life.

However, this wretched time of illness changed all that.
While agonizingly painful, it became, for me, a Light FROM the Darkness,

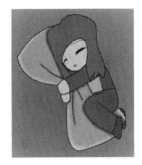

The story that ensues in this book shows how going through this darkness of pain and illness changed my life, turning me into a healer of maladies, of anxiety, and of whatever ails a person.

Chana Klein

You will read how I came to understand
what most of us go through while suffering,
how I got to figure out the mechanisms of
illness & healing, and how to apply that to
help another.

Rabbi Maimon Directs Me to Be a Healer

It all began in 1993 when I met with Kabbalist, Rabbi Eliyahu Maimon, recommended by Rabbi Simcha Weinberg.

"You have healing hands. You have to release the power to heal from your hands," Rabbi Maimon told me.

Then again in 1995, as soon as I was entering the room we were to meet in, Rabbi Maimon, looking at me, said the same words.

Chana Klein

Without my sharing with him any details
about my life or family, he told me the
Hebrew initials of my youngest son's name,
who had been very ill years before.

He told me it was my hands that healed my
son. (I imagine he meant directed by the
Almighty.)

Brett often asked from his sick bed, that I
put my hands on his back. "Rub," he would
say.
And so, even when Brett was not conscious,
I kept my hands on him, knowing it was
what felt best to him.

Light FROM the Darkness of Illness
& Physical Disability

"You must heal people,"

Rabbi Maimon told me on both visits.

"You have to release the power to heal from

your hands," he repeated.

Very content with my career as a teacher, I

did not understand the rabbi's message.

I quickly forgot the directions he had given

me to do things, spiritual things, like pray at

a body of water, kiss the mezuzah, etc.,

having had neither interest in, nor

understanding of, healing in the first place.

But, clearly, God had other plans for me.

Chana Klein

In 1995, I was going through an increasingly horrific experience of being harassed at work, which intensified with time.

I loved the classroom and my precious students.

But the harassment from the administration was extremely intrusive.
It caused me to have to be on alert all the time.

Early one March morning in 1997, under great stress, I stood at the large window of my classroom.

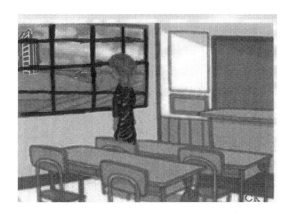

Looking toward Heaven, I requested of God, "Get me out of here!"

Right after my prayer, I walked down the flight of steps that I had descended so many times, every day that school year.

Chana Klein

This time I was heading to my car to get the additional bag which contained the teaching materials that I had created at home the day before.

Unusual for my athletic body, I missed a step, landing on what was now my twisted ankle.
Unable to put any weight on that ankle, I couldn't get up.

The hospital emergency room's diagnosis of a broken ankle that day, led to an orthopedic doctor's diagnosis of Reflex Sympathetic Dystrophy (RSD) one week later, after a positive tri-phase bone scan.

Light FROM the Darkness of Illness & Physical Disability

By the following year, the RSD illness
spread throughout my body, until I was
diagnosed with "Full-Body RSD."

The torturous pain of RSD and my previous
adverse reaction to every medication that I
had ever tried, led me to searching for relief
through alternative methods.

So, my journey to becoming a healer began
with healing myself.

I searched for a healer who would touch me
and take it all away.
That's all I wanted.

Chana Klein

For years, I had ignored and forgotten
Rabbi Maimon's urging me to be a healer
myself.

But my life was now changed.
Now I *had* to learn to heal, no matter what
other plans I had for my life.

The search for relief from the incredible,
agonizing, throbbing, from the numbness,
the burning and the freezing pain of RSD,
was on.

Light FROM the Darkness of Illness & Physical Disability

The sleepless nights and the lack of any moments of relief from the pain were truly unbearable.

Yes, the search was on.

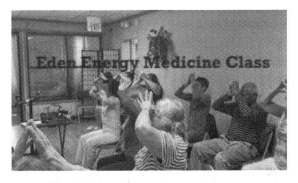

I attended many seminars, classes, programs.

One led to the other.

Chana Klein

I undertook trainings in many healing modalities, all at the same time.
I learned each, and learned it well.

Most importantly, I learned that healing is a process.
Healing is not the "event" I was in search of.

As I continued doing the things I was learning, I did get some relief.
While I was learning alternative healing, I still went to Dr. Hooshmand, the RSD guru in Florida, who injected my spine with what felt like a huge quantity of steroids.

But, the steroids in my system did not allow me to sleep, not even a short nap.

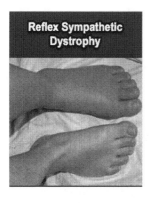

It did give me some short-term temporary relief from the pain though.

When Dr. Hooshmand's injections wore off within a few weeks, it felt awful again.

At that time, the pain would return even stronger, or so it felt.

Chana Klein

Many Teachers, Many Masters

I went from one seminar to another where various modalities of healing were taught.

Rosalyn L. Bruyere was one of my first teachers.
I am so grateful to Rosalyn for introducing me to the concept of energy.
She was the first to teach me how to feel energy, how to move it, and how to use it to heal another.

33

Light FROM the Darkness of Illness
& Physical Disability

I learned with Rosalyn for about five years,
following her seminars around the country,
and then privately in her home in
California.

After several years, Rosalyn advised me to
go out to study with other teachers, for I
had grasped her teachings well.

I then learned with two of her students who
developed and taught Nervous System
Energy Work (NSEW.)

I found NSEW invaluable for me and for
my clients.

I continue to use the techniques with my
clients.

Chana Klein

I took other courses online with several
organizations.

But I learn better in person.

However, before that awareness, I took an
online course with NICABM.
I was torturously bored with the teacher on
the recording.

Eden Energy Medicine /
Innersource

The book that the NICABM teacher was using was that of Donna Eden, rather than her own book.

So rather than continue being bored, I made a call to Innersource, the office headquarters of Donna Eden.

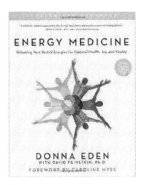

The following week, I was attending a seminar in Florida, learning in person with Donna Eden herself.

Chana Klein

It was 2003 when I began learning with Donna, following her to every course she was teaching, before there was a certification program for Innersource.

Eventually, many years and courses later, I had completed all the certifications Innersource offers, up to Advanced Practitioner, proficient in working with Grid and Regression.

The Eden Energy
Medicine (EEM)
modalities and
techniques,
Donna's work and
her instructors,
have been
marvelous and life
changing.

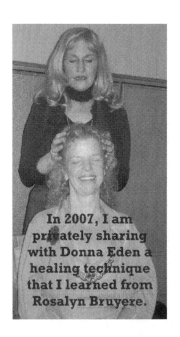

In 2007, I am
privately sharing
with Donna Eden a
healing technique
that I learned from
Rosalyn Bruyere.

EEM techniques
have had a great deal to do with my total
healing of RSD and of so many other
conditions, physical, emotional, and
spiritual.

Chana Klein

It is 2017 as I am writing this.

I still do EEM work most days on myself
and with clients, lifesaving and life-giving
work for sure.

My gratitude to Donna Eden, her husband
David Feinstein, and her staff, is endless.
To this day, I continue to attend their
trainings and to expand my healing
abilities.

With EEM, I have learned, and had endless
practice in, all nine systems of Chinese
Medicine, how to use them practically to
balance my energy and that of my clients.

Light FROM the Darkness of Illness & Physical Disability

I have learned to be a healing detective and to test and find the source of my client's problem and how to fix it.

EEM has turned me into an almost magician, able to heal maladies like Cancer, RSD, Multiple Sclerosis, Mental Illness, Emotional Problems, Depression, Panic, Trauma, and just about every illness that walks in the door.

I cannot, in this writing, share the whole of what EEM has given me.

Chana Klein

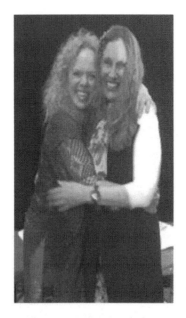

Donna Eden and me at EEM for Animals Oct 2017

Just know that I am beyond grateful.

Neuro Emotional Technique
(NET)

In 2004, at an American Academy of Pain Management (AAPM) conference, I was introduced to a miraculously effective modality, Neuro Emotional Technique (NET). NET is a lifesaving, life-giving modality that I use every day in almost every session.

This technique has also turned me into a healing magician of all maladies.

I never cease to be completely enraptured as I continue to attend the expansive NET seminars, because the learning and development of this modality is endless.

It just gets deeper and better as its creator Dr. Scott Walker, DC and NET manager, Dr. Deb Walker, DC dedicatedly work on expanding it and sharing it with us, the NET practitioners.

Light FROM the Darkness of Illness
& Physical Disability

NET heals the stress, the emotional
component of every illness, every trauma,
every bad memory, disturbing dream, pain,
disability, etc.

NET facilitates our finding where and when
the illness process began on each client.

All illness begins with the emotions, the
Neuro Emotional Complex (NEC).
An NEC may be defined as an unresolved
stress pattern which creates neurological
and physiological imbalances.

Chana Klein

I am convinced, from my experience in
healing myself and others, that to
completely heal, so that the illness never
returns, we must clear the emotions that
precipitated and extended the illness.

I do that for my clients through NET.
When I deal only with the symptoms
without working on the underlying
emotions, the illness invariably returns.
It is essential to get to the original event
that planted the seeds for the illness,
and to clear the Neuro Emotional

Component (NEC), in order to achieve complete, real, enduring healing.

We learn, in the NET seminars, to locate the NEC, to find its original event, where and when it began, and to clear it from the body.

I have seen that one session of NET is more effective than years of therapy in getting the results my clients are in search of.

NET is invaluable.

Chana Klein

It has changed my life.

Really, it has healed my life, and the lives of endless clients, clearing everything that ever bothered me, and them.

I am so grateful to Dr. Scott Walker and Dr. Deb Walker for gifting me with their incredible healing modality, for being there at all times to respond to my questions, with such patience and such love.

Light FROM the Darkness of Illness
& Physical Disability

Through the practice of NET, I have
been able to reach my own truth and
have guided my clients to reaching
theirs.

NET assists in our becoming free to be
who we are, not who we think we
should be.

That is Real Healing.

I am so blessed to be in the NET Family
of learning incredible healing.

Other Trainings

I continue to attend NET seminars, EEM trainings, and to deepen my learning with a gifted Doctor of Chinese Medicine, Melanie Smith (WellWithin.org), who teaches small classes based in EEM and Chinese Medicine to Advanced EEM practitioners.

We learn the greater depths of Chinese Medicine and additional techniques to increase immunity, brain function, healing of cancer, heart issues and so much more to serve our clients.

I graduated other programs such as The Academy for Guided Imagery, also a meaningful training.

I trained, also, in Korean Hand Therapy (KHT), in the Handle Program (Holistic Approach to Neuro Development and Learning Efficiency) and privately, with Judith Bluestone, the founder and creator of HANDLE.

In addition, I graduated many coaching programs, achieving endless certifications in General coaching, ADHD coaching, Family coaching, Recovery coaching, too many to mention, but my favorite being ADD Coach Academy (ADDCA) founded and taught by David Giwerc, MCC.

My trainings gave me the basis to develop my own techniques for working with those diagnosed with Autism, Asperger's, Schizophrenia,

OCD, Tourette's, and a multitude of mental disabilities.

For more on that, read my next book: *Light FROM the Darkness of Invisible Disability &Disorder: True Stories of Understanding & Recovery from Learning Disability, ADHD, Autism, & Other Brain/Body Wirings*.

I have created and teach a training for coaches called *Coaching the Uncoachable*, in which I share how to work with clients who seem to be not workable, but who really are the most wonderful to work with, once we know how.

Man Plans and God Laughs

I was a dedicated teacher for 34 years,
never, ever wanting to change
careers.
Then, my life circumstances changed
my career *for* me.

There is a saying in Yiddish "Der *mentch*
trakht un Got lakht."
It means "Man plans and God laughs."
I never would have imagined how
enriched my life would be as a Real
Healer, how much I would learn, how it
would expand my mind and my being,

nor how healing and empowering it

would be for me to know all that I do

now.

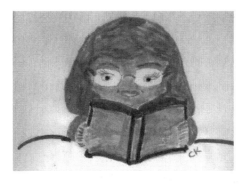

And the learning never ends . . .

INTRODUCTION

I wrote this book for the myriad of us who have coped with, and are still coping with, illness and/or disability, our own, and/or that of someone close to us.

You will read in this book many stories of how I learned to heal myself and others from many illnesses and disabilities.

This is a book of stories to understand illness, why it occurs, why it continues, and what gets it better.

Light FROM the Darkness of Illness & Physical Disability

I healed my own Stage IV Ovarian Cancer nine years ago (as of this writing), my Reflex Sympathetic Dystrophy, my Candida, my Interstitial Cystitis, my numerous bone issues, hormonal issues, heart issues, anxiety, panic, addiction, endless health issues, and paralyzing learning disabilities of ADHD, Dyslexia, Dyscalculia, et al.

Having healed myself, and having healed hundreds of clients, with God's help, I am convinced that almost all illness begins with emotions, stress, and what we are feeling before its onset.

Chana Klein

In my first book, *Light FROM the Darkness: A Different Perspective on Difficult Times,* I share my story of having been hurt in so many ways, especially by those who were supposed to take care of me.

I believe that my childhood emotional trauma and physical abuse led to the inordinate amount of physical and emotional illnesses and disabilities I had as a teen and an adult.

It led to my having had to heal myself of each of the issues mentioned in this book. I have suffered them all.

Light FROM the Darkness of Illness
& Physical Disability

I have healed myself of each, with God's help.

In my work as a healer, I find that all illness and disability begin with shock, trauma, and negative emotions.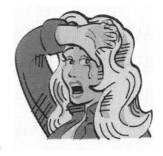

The foundation of much of my work with clients has everything to do with having them face themselves and find their own Light FROM the Darkness.

Chana Klein

The challenge in writing a book about

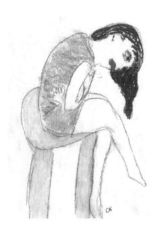

illness and

disability is to put

into words how

devastating it feels

to be ill, to be

disabled, to be in

pain,

be it physically,

mentally, emotionally, or spiritually, be it a

learning disability, an addiction,

or any state of being that renders us to be

less than who we can be.

After the fact, when the pain is gone, when

the recovery has taken place, it's easy to

look back and romanticize the times of illness.

I can easily make it all sound so glorious having already been healed.

But the stories in this book, while they explain healing, do not get lost in the glory of having been healed.

The stories re-live how dark it feels to be ill, while acknowledging the great lessons learned from that darkness, and of course, explaining how we get better.

Chana Klein

Thus, the *Light FROM the Darkness of Illness*
& Physical Disability.

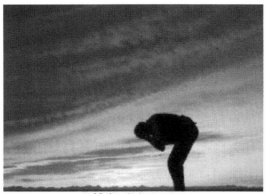

publicdomainpictures.net

Understanding illness and healing is as
complex as understanding the human
psyche and systems.

Light FROM the Darkness of Illness
& Physical Disability

For example, some of the stories in *Light FROM the Darkness of Illness & Physical Disability* explain how the illness experience offers benefits that we may not be aware of, but that can keep us ill.

Even though it feels devastating, illness is not as simple and clear as one would think.

This book is for those in search of understanding what makes us ill, what keeps us ill, and how to heal, be it mentally, emotionally, physically, spiritually. . . be it an illness, a physical disability, a learning disability, an addiction, or any other kind of state that needs recovery.

Two Books

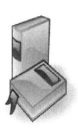 Because I had so many stories and so much information to share about healing, the book became too long.

Therefore, I divided it into two books:

1. *Light FROM the Darkness of Illness and Physical Disability: What Makes Us Ill, What Keeps Us Ill, & How to Heal*

2. *Light FROM the Darkness of Invisible Disability & Disorder:*

Light FROM the Darkness of Illness & Physical Disability

*True Stories of Understanding &
Recovery from Learning Disability,
ADHD, Autism, and other Brain/Body
Wirings.*

So, this book explains what makes us ill,
what keeps us ill, and how to heal, from
physical illness, while the next book deals
with disabilities that others can't see.

The books are written also for those who
relate to, or care for, people in any condition
of illness or disability.
They too will gain from reading the stories
and from learning the lessons of these
books.

Chana Klein

My Definition of Illness & Disability

Disability and illness here are defined as whatever stops us from being who we can be.

These conditions of illness and disability rob us of our potential.

Reviving Our Lost Potential

The stories in this book are about what creates healing and how to revive our lost potential.

Light FROM the Darkness of Illness & Physical Disability

I, the author, have experienced the darkness 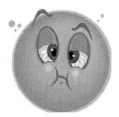 of feeling too ill to get up, to lift my head, to talk to anyone, to answer the phone, to keep my eyes open, or to think clearly.

I have been the recipient of endless, hopeless diagnoses from many physicians, all illnesses and disabilities from which I have been fully restored.

I spent much of my childhood needing crutches to walk, after having been a battered child.

Chana Klein

As an adult, I became disabled once again, for an additional 22 years, unable to ambulate without crutches, until I found Real Healing.

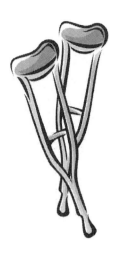

In the interim, I was stricken with various acute, chronic, life-threatening illnesses, diseases, disabilities and addictions.

Does Illness Help Us?

In search of healing, I became aware of aspects of what each illness did, not only *to* me, but *for* me.

Yes, sometimes the illness we get helps us in some way.

I call that *"The Benefit of the Illness."* (See the story that follows.)

Chana Klein

The benefit we get from an illness makes the illness more difficult to let go of and to heal from.

Illness and healing are complicated because we, as human beings, are complicated in how we think and feel.

We often don't understand, or are not aware of, what is happening within ourselves that creates illness, or of what creates healing.

In this book, you will learn about healing from a different perspective than what is popular, even in healing circles.

Light FROM the Darkness of Illness & Physical Disability

For example, you will see, in this book, that the effort to think positively is rarely helpful, unless it is a natural progression of thought.

(For more on this, see chapter: *The Truth About Thinking Positively.*)

Facing your darkness brings you to the Light that is from the *real* you.

It is the Light FROM the Darkness that fills each of us.

Facing our darkness brings us to the Light we are in search of.

Reading the stories in this book and the next book, will help you gain a real understanding of how to find your own *Light FROM the Darkness of Illness & Disability*.

Find out how to unlock your potential and how to find Real Healing.

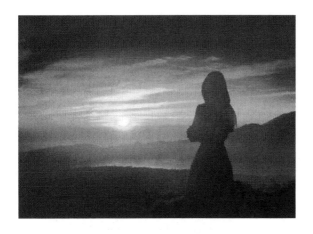

Staring straight into the Darkness removes its terrifying power.

What remains is great Light.

Chana Klein

STORIES OF UNDERSTANDING AND OVERCOMING ILLNESS & PHYSICAL DISABILITY

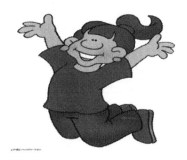

The Benefit of the Illness

(Why We Remain Ill)

*How many of us actually find what
we are in search of?*

*Then, once we find it, what do we do
with it?*

W hy is it that some people just do not
get better?

Chana Klein

Why (at the time of my writing this story)
do I still use crutches to walk?

There are people who go from one healer to
another, searching for an answer.
They *say* they want to get better.
They *think* they want to get better.

How many of us are searching in that way?

How many of us are seeking the truth for
ourselves, or for someone else, like a child, a
parent, or a friend?

How many of us are searching for the truth of how to live, of what to do, or what to think?

How many of us actually find what we are in search of? But then, once we find it, what do we do with it? Do we change according to the truth we have found?

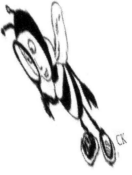

Some client stories (not the real names)

Marie:

*Being excused from what we think we
have to do, is a benefit of an illness.*

I ask Marie, a 4th stage cancer patient:
"What will you miss about having cancer
when we get you better?"

She readily answers:

"I will miss being free of the responsibility
of taking care of my daughter-in-law's
house and children. The fact that I am sick,
excuses me from going over there."

It amazed her further that the kids are still

well and thriving . . .

and the house is fine . . .

even though she had not been there during

the past two years of her illness.

Being excused from what we think we have

to do, is a benefit of an illness.

Harold:

*While Harold wanted a friend so very
much, the benefit of not having a friend
had been winning.*

Harold has never had a friend.

78

Chana Klein

We all need a friend, someone to speak with
and to share with.
You would think that not having a friend is
a terrible thing.
And it is.

But with that is also the benefit.

I asked Harold, "When you get a friend,
what will you miss about *not* having a
friend?"
Harold, who is on the autism spectrum,
talks in bullet points.
From the tip of his tongue, he shot out a list
of at least 20 things that he will miss about

not having a friend when he finally does get
a friend.

Among what he will miss was the complete
control he feels he has when he is alone.

He will also miss the freedom to avoid
conflict because, to him, conflict is so
unpleasant.

He said also that in having a friend, he will
miss the feeling of not having any
obligations.

Harold shared so much more about what he
will miss about not having a friend.

While Harold wanted a friend so very
much, the benefit of *not* having a friend had
been winning.

Not having a friend meant he would have
no conflict, no obligations, and more control
of his life.
He was reluctant to give these up.

That is, until based on his new awareness,
he made an inner decision.

His new awareness was a realization of
what he really wants.

A person who stays in a situation, even if it's awful, usually chooses to do so from the bottom of his soul.

Yet, in his actions, he may keep seeking to find an answer.

Yitro's story

He (Yitro) is in his glory, now having found the truth that he has been seeking his entire life.

We meet a "seeker" in The Torah portion that is named after him.

Yitro, the father-in-law of Moshe (Moses),
hears about God Splitting the Red Sea and
about the War with Amalek that God
fought for the Israelites
(Rashi, Exodus 18:1).

He also hears the same news that everyone
hears about the Revelation at Sinai.

So, Yitro travels with Moshe's wife and
children to join the Jewish people and to be
a part of these phenomenal events.

Yitro is a seeker.

He seeks and searches

for truth.

The commentaries share

with us how Yitro has tried

multiple religions and forms of

worship.

He is in his glory now, having found the

truth that he has been seeking his entire life.

That truth that Yitro found is in Torah from

Sinai.

He declares, "Now I know that Hashem

(God), is greater than all the gods."

Chana Klein

(Exodus 18:11)

But what does Yitro, who is a seer and a

seeker, do with the truth that he has found?

Does he now live according to that truth?

Does he finally stop searching other

religions and start learning the depth of The

Torah?

The Book of Numbers reveals what Yitro

did with the truth he found.

Moshe asks Yitro to come with the Israelites

on their journey to the promised land.

> "Go with us and we shall treat you well,
> for God has spoken of good for Israel."
> (Numbers 10:29)

Light FROM the Darkness of Illness & Physical Disability

But Yitro, even though he knows that he
found his truth with the Israelites, responds
that he will not go with them.
Rather, he will return to his native land and
his family. (Numbers 10:29)

In other words, Yitro declares that he will
go back to his old life, ignoring his great
find.

Moshe continues to try to convince Yitro to
follow the truth that he has found.
(Numbers 10:31)
But to no avail.

Chana Klein

For Yitro, after having sought and tried
every other religion for most of his life,
finding Truth in The Torah from Sinai, must
have been an awesome moment for him.

To finally find what he had been searching
for all his life. Wow!
For any of us, it would be amazing to find
what we have been searching for.

But are we any different from Yitro?
What do we do with those answers when
we find them?

Do we internalize the truth that we find and
change our ways?

Or . . .

Do we go back to our old ways, as Yitro does?

Do we ignore what we have found and keep searching?

There are those who seek and search but do not do anything with the answers they find.

They go back to seeking.

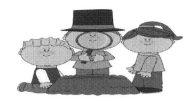

Why Do We Ignore the Healing That We Find?

The Benefit

For many, there is a benefit to staying where we are and just continuing the search for an answer.

There is a benefit in the discomfort of our condition.

Why would anyone do that? Why would a person hold onto his illness or onto anything negative in his life?

I have found that, for many of us, there is a benefit to staying where we are and just continuing the search for an answer.

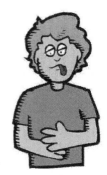

There is a benefit in the discomfort of our condition.

There is a benefit to the illness.

Robert:

Robert called me from a California hospital to heal his heart condition.
He was only 38 years old.

I asked him, "What will you miss about this heart problem when we get you better?" I ask many of my clients how their suffering is helping them in some way.

It amazes me that the answer is often so readily available to them.

Robert's heart condition rose up when he realized that his parents, who live in Argentina, are aging.

He remembered worrying that they may need financial help soon and that he would

have to use his own money to support
them.

Robert is a planner.
He plans for every
penny.

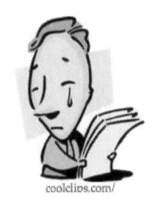

cooldips.com/

The benefit to Robert
of being in the
hospital with a heart problem is that no one
would expect any kind of financial help
from him, while he is in this condition.

While Robert loves his parents, deep down,
his illness was of great benefit to him in that

he believed it would save him from the
financial loss of helping his parents.

Just the same, he knew this was not how he
wanted to be.

We found alternative ways to deal with his
worry about finances and with his need to
plan ahead for every penny.

In our work together, he realized how
impossible it is to plan for everything that
will happen.

The result? His heart condition became a
thing of the past shortly after that.

Susan:

Susan was diagnosed schizophrenic as a

teenager.

At the beginning of our work together, she

was plagued with daily hallucinations.

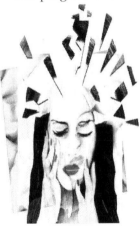

Susan is a very high

soul, as I have found

all schizophrenics to

be. They strive to be

good.

Susan wanted very

much to think of

herself as "sweet and good."

There was always a logic to the
hallucinations she was experiencing.

When Susan had a thought that she felt did
not make her "sweet and good" (the way
she wanted herself to be,) she simply had
the figure appear in the hallucination saying
the thought, as if it did not belong to Susan.
For example, "Mary Smith said my mother
is bad."
This hallucination makes no sense until one
understands Susan's way of thinking.

While Susan loved her mother, part of her
was angry with her, largely because of the
treatments she was put through as a teen
and as an adult to deal with her
schizophrenia.
But Susan did not want to own the fact that
she could be a person who has anger.
Susan wanted to have only "sweet and
good" thoughts.

So, she would give that anger to the figure
she was hallucinating, Mary Smith.
Then, the thought would not be Susan's.
It was now the thought of Mary Smith.

Susan, now, could blame the anger on someone else and remain the person she wants to think she is, the one who is "sweet and good."

There was great benefit to Susan in her private hallucinatory world which was never boring.

Owning the feelings as her own, rather than those of the characters of her hallucinations, has greatly relieved the occurrence of her hallucinations.

Susan received so much relief from looking at the reality, and at her patterns of thought, that she married and gave birth to children, whom she is raising with help from her husband and her family.

To Each Illness, There Is a Benefit.

Each illness serves a specific purpose for those of us who suffer from it.
If the illness persists, then we likely need that illness for something more important to us than getting better.

It might be an excuse for failure.

It could be our
subconscious
way of getting
others to care for
us.

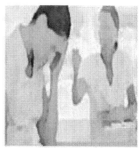

Image Source: wearandcheer.com

It might be for the special attention we
receive, or it could be a way to get a
reprieve from being criticized, which is also
an outcome of being ill.

In order to get better, we need to be aware
of what that benefit is.

My Story

As a mind-body practitioner who heals so many maladies of others and of my own, I had to examine why I still used crutches to walk.

I had to do my own searching.

By 1997 I was diagnosed with Reflex Sympathetic Dystrophy (RSD.)
I was in horrific pain, and very embarrassed that I needed crutches, after having been a skilled athlete.

Chana Klein

The first two years of being stricken with
RSD, I was pretty much homebound.

When I began coming back into the world
and even presented on stage at conferences,
I noticed that people were nice to me.

I realized that people want to help a person
who is disabled.

It was so healing, not just of RSD, but of my
whole life, to have people want to help me,
to have people being kind to me.

How healing it is to have so many run to
hold the door for me, even though I know I
could push it open and fly right through by
myself.

Just the fact that
they would
want to is
healing to me.

How healing it is to go on stage, and rather
than see daggers of jealousy thrown at me
from the audience's faces, seeing people on
the edge of their seats ready to help me,

Chana Klein

ready to
support,
totally
rooting for
my success.

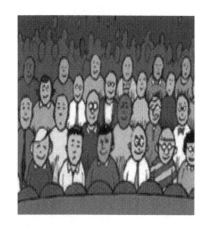

On
crutches, I
am no longer a threat to anyone, for no one
wants to be me.

No one wants to be a person who uses
crutches to walk, a person who needs to
accommodate how she does everything, in
order to do what everyone else does with
ease.

It is the benefit of the illness that I am not
ready to give up.

I am not ready to face the
world without the shield of
using crutches.

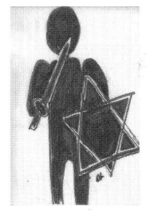

My crutches are my Shield
of David, protecting me
from the worst side of
people and bringing out their best, for
people like to help one who they think
needs it.

Behind these crutches, I can have an
encyclopedic knowledge of nutrition,

healing, coaching, Torah, and a host of other subjects.

I can be an intuitive without anyone being jealous.

I can be me without the suppressive force of those who want to attack me, because when I am behind those crutches, no one wants to.

So, too, for Yitro, there is a benefit, I am sure, in continuing to be a seeker without living up to what he has found.

Light FROM the Darkness of Illness & Physical Disability

Perhaps the great responsibility of a Torah life, a life of commitment, or even of a role of leadership in such a nation, was too much to imagine, had he internalized and committed to what he had found.

There are many benefits we each have in not internalizing and changing, according to the truth we have found.

But in order to get better, in order to heal, in order to change, we need to understand the benefit we are getting from being where we are.

We need to be aware of that before we can take on the benefit of being who we want to be.

Knowing the benefit of our illness unlocks the key to the jail that we put ourselves in.

Then we can be free to decide, to heal, and to be the person we choose to be.

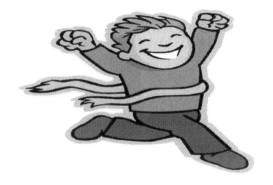

<u>Post Script 2016</u> - Years after writing this story, I am free of my need for crutches mentally, emotionally, and physically.
I accomplished this healing by doing what I write about in this book.

More details surrounding the progress that took place are in a story in one of my next books.

I must add, here, that after letting go of my crutches, people are *still* nice to me.

What an amazing surprise!!!!

Chana Klein

REAL HEALING - THINKING ABOUT IT DIFFERENTLY

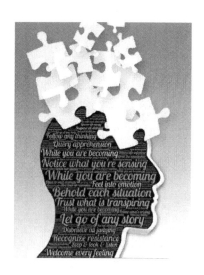

The Truth about "Positive" Thinking

I have heard well-meaning friends say: "You need to think positive. "

But I have found that the effort to think positively is rarely helpful, unless it is a natural progression of thought.

Rather, the *effort* to think positively becomes repressive.

It often causes guilt
feelings if the person
feels s/he is not doing
it well.
Guilt feelings make
us ill.

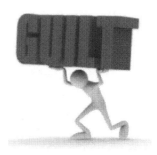

Contrary to what most think, in dealing
with grief, sadness, anger, or any other
stuck feeling, it is important to allow oneself
to truly feel those feelings.

Attempting to think positively prevents us
from facing our darkness, which is where
Real Healing begins.

Light FROM the Darkness of Illness & Physical Disability

The truth is that we need to first feel our dark feelings and to face them before we can come anywhere close to thinking positively.

Trying to *force* ourselves to feel what we don't genuinely feel, takes up the time and energy that we could be feeling our real feelings, and begin our Real Healing.

A person who is repressing emotions is creating "stuck" energy, a Chinese medicine term that indicates the opposite of healthy energy flow.
The aim of healing work is to create flow and balance.

Emotions and energy, when blocked or stuck, cause emotional and physical problems.

Stuck energy is caused by refusing to acknowledge feelings, by being in denial about them, by substituting one emotion for another.

For example, feeling anger when the real emotion might be fear, or feeling gratitude when the real emotion is anger, causes stuck energy in the body.

These stuck states cause illness, disability and other problems.

It is most healing to feel what we honestly

feel, rather than what we *think* we should

feel.

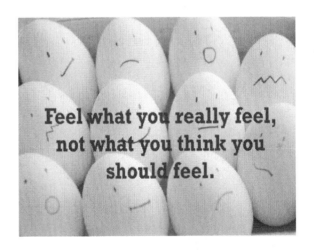

Linda

I have discovered the truth about trying to be positive through my work with clients like Linda.

Linda met with her oncologist, her mom sitting next to her.
Linda sensed the oncologist's concern before she even heard his words.

Most of the words he said were a blur to Linda.

All that registered for her, all she really
heard, was the doctor's diagnosis: "Stage
IIIC Breast Cancer."

At home, her mom who loves her so dearly,
sat on the foot of her bed and told her to
think positively.

How many of us hear that advice from well-
meaning friends and relatives?

"Think positively!" they tell us, as if it were
the deepest wisdom.
As if it were so easy!
"Think positively and it will be fine."

Chana Klein

Linda tries to be positive.

She tries to not think those scared thoughts.

In her effort to think positively, the terror

she feels over her Stage IIIC Cancer

diagnosis is not faced.

Linda repeats the words "it will be fine,"

trying to force them into her psyche.

But the message, "It will be fine," does not

serve to make her feel better.

Neither does it help in minimizing the

disease process, or its effects on her body

> What happens when people open their
> hearts? They get better.
> Harumk Murakami, Norwegian Wood

Linda's First Session

L inda comes to our first session.

She cries that she is a failure -

a failure because she is failing to think

positively.

Now, Linda is suffering not only from her
illness and from hearing her diagnosis,
but added is the guilt she feels for failing to
think positively, as others have told her to
do.

The effort to think positively, besides
repressing her real feelings, is adding to her
illness.

So how does this work?
When we try to think positively, we are
forever fighting what we really feel.

We keep fighting our darkness.

Light FROM the Darkness of Illness & Physical Disability

Our attempt to think positively involves refusing to look at that darkness.

We are trying to replace our darkness with happy thoughts that are not, at the time, really ours, rather than embracing the thoughts and feelings that are real and truly our own.

We turn away from our real thoughts because it's too uncomfortable and scary to face what we honestly feel.

But, pushing our real feelings away doesn't work because the thoughts we try so hard to extinguish, never go away.

Chana Klein

The darkness we are trying to push away
becomes more and more stuck in our
system, as we resist that darkness.

The effort towards positive thinking is so
much work.
It leads us to frustration, repression, guilt
feelings, and endless illness.

In addition, the struggle to think positively
suppresses our symptoms in the same way
that medication does.

Medication masks symptoms but does not
treat the source of the illness.

That is why people have to stay on a drug for so long, sometimes indefinitely, or the symptoms return.

Medications are often ineffective or trigger more problems than they solve.

Linda learned that it is more healing for her to just "be" who she really is and feel what she really feels, rather than to struggle trying to be who she is not.

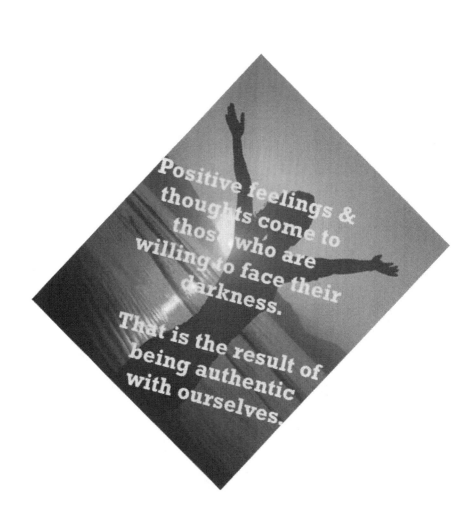

Positive feelings &
thoughts come to
those who are
willing to face their
darkness.

That is the result of
being authentic
with ourselves.

Unshed Tears

I have been asked if facing one's darkness can lead to depression.

Feeling one's feelings can, of course, lead to some sadness and even to crying.
But that is not depression.

Depression is a treatable mental illness with many more symptoms than an unhappy mood.

Medical researchers have found that depression is caused by biology, by neurotransmitters, by genes, and other theories.

It has never been believed that depression is from feeling real feelings.

According to Traditional Chinese Medicine (TCM), crying is very healthy, as is feeling authentic sadness.

There is a condition in Chinese medicine known as "Unshed Tears."

In other words, NOT letting oneself feel or cry when needed, stops the body's flow and causes stuck feelings, resulting in stuck

energy.

This stuck energy shows as bags under the

eyes.

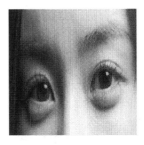 Those bags are
called "Unshed
Tears" in Chinese
Medicine.

Unshed Tears show on the face as thick

bags under the eyes.

Unshed Tears also indicate that there is a

kidney problem.

Chana Klein

Facing one's darkness and authentically
crying could help alleviate Unshed Tears.

If that person lets himself feel his feelings
and cry, he may release those bags.

Crying is healthy for the human system.

Facing one's darkness does not cause
depression.

Dark cures dark.

It does not create more darkness.

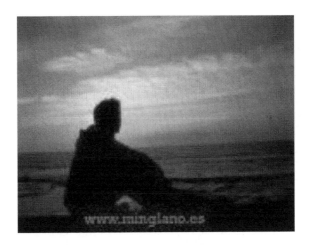

Doing it Differently

Linda experienced how *forcing* positive thoughts on herself was not helpful.
She realized it was not productive for her to *try* to "think positively."
The attempt to feel what she does not naturally feel created incongruity in the systems of her body.

The *effort* to think positively does not heal.
It harms.

Light FROM the Darkness of Illness & Physical Disability

The Light that she found by facing her darkness, is from her real feelings, and is from the real Linda.
It is from her authentic feelings.

It is the Light FROM the Darkness that fills each of us with healing.

Facing our darkness, our pain, our suffering, brings us to the Light we are in search of.

Facing our darkness facilitates our body and our mind to heal.

It energizes our healing vitality into action.

Facing one's darkness creates a Healing Response.

Facing the feelings of our suffering animates the part of our spirit that heals us.

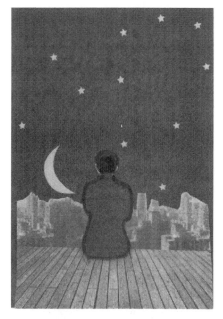

In fact, it is the key to healing.

Light FROM the Darkness of Illness & Physical Disability

I have experienced it personally many
times.
I have been writing about it and using it in
my healing work for years.

But of course, it doesn't make sense that
when I look into the darkness, I end up
experiencing great light, or any light at all.

I would never have thought of such an
outrageous idea, had I not felt the healing
that I experienced so powerfully that I
could not avoid it.

Nor could I avoid the light that I got.

> **Our wounds are often the openings into the best and most beautiful part of us.**
> **David Richo**

"Like Cures Like" . . .

And my own take on this: "Dark cures Dark"

"Dark Cures Dark" is further explained with a healing principle known as "Like Cures Like."

What Is the Science Behind "Like Cures Like?"

Hippocrates, the Father of Medicine, who lived from 460 to 370 BCE, taught:

> "By similar things a disease is produced, and through the application of the like, is cured."

That means that to get better, we need to reproduce what made us ill.

We need to face it and focus on it.

Yoni

Let's illustrate this with the example of 4-year-old Yoni.

Yoni is the center of attention in his family of himself and his parents.

He gets the attention he needs whenever he wants it.

He lives happily with his toys and the attention of his family.
One day, Yoni's parents bring home his new-born brother.

135

Now, this little intruder is in his mother's

lap all the

time,

which

used to

belong to

Yoni.

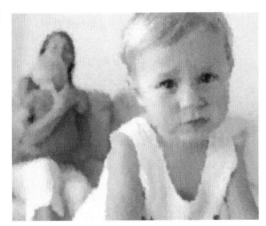

All

visitors are looking at the baby.

No one is interested in Yoni anymore.

Yoni is not happy.

He wants to send the baby back.

But his parents seem to love the new baby

and plan to keep him.

It may be that Yoni's parents love Yoni as much as ever, and that this is all just in Yoni's mind.

But this is Yoni's "Emotional Reality" and in order to clear it, it must be treated as if it is true, at least for Yoni.

Eventually, the acute pain of the intrusion that Yoni has experienced from the arrival of his new brother fades in the background, and Yoni goes on with his life.

Until . . . Yoni is in 5th grade and the children are assigned learning partners.

Light FROM the Darkness of Illness & Physical Disability

Yoni's best friend, Alan, is learning with
another classmate.

Yoni is feeling terrible.
He feels jealousy that is way out of
proportion to what is normal.

This is because he never processes (or faces)
the pain that he had felt as a 4-year old.

That pain settles in one of his body organs,
ready to come out when a similar situation
arises.

Yoni has not had an opportunity to face his
suffering over the intrusion.

He does not try to process and clear it by facing how it disturbed him.

So, the event and its emotions become stuck in Yoni's physiology.

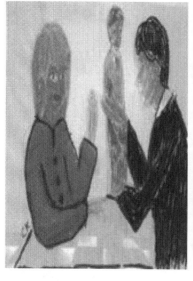

Then, at age 17, Yoni is in love with Jessica, whom he sees talking with an acquaintance. The insecurity he feels takes him over. It feels almost unbearable.

Light FROM the Darkness of Illness & Physical Disability

Yoni needs to clear from his system what happened when he was 4-years-old, as well as what followed, in order to be okay.

All these events are connected by the same energy pathway, the energy pathway that deals with feelings of abandonment, insecurity, and jealousy.

All this can be cleared by facing and re-experiencing that darkness-event that happened when he was 4, the arrival of his baby brother.

Yoni would need to focus on the event and re-feel it, while he holds certain acupressure

points, which will help him to process his
feelings.

(Acupressure points are connected to
specific emotions. When held, they can clear
blockages in meridians where energy
flows.)

Feeling joy, sadness and anger are all
perfectly normal experiences that we have
in our day-to-day lives.
It is when these emotions become excessive,
or are repressed, and turned inward, that
they can cause disease.

Light FROM the Darkness of Illness & Physical Disability

One of the reasons that keeping our emotions locked up inside can have negative effects on our physical health is that they remain stuck inside of our bodies.

That stuckness can lead to a blockage of blood and a blockage of energy flow. This leads to disease.

But Yoni does not yet have any idea that such a thing exists and so does not do anything to clear it.

So, at age 25, he develops circulation problems, as well as burning in the soles of his feet.

These symptoms can be traced to the same energy pathway as those original feelings of insecurity.

This energy pathway has developed what NET calls a "Neuro Emotional Complex" (NEC).
These are stuck emotions that need to be processed.

And those emotions can be traced to the original event of Yoni getting a new brother.

It can all be easily cleared in a session with an NET practitioner.

Then, Yoni may go on with his life free of those stuck physical and emotional issues, and their physical manifestations.

In the NET session, Yoni needs to re-experience the original suffering in a controlled way, face it, process it, and then he will be fine.

> We are healed of suffering only by experiencing it to the full.
> — Marcel Proust

What Yoni Did

Yoni remained stuck in his pattern of jealousy and insecurity and was powerless over it until he processed the original event and the Neuro Emotional Complex attached to it, that is, the birth of his brother.

For Yoni, once he got help having that done, it was like a miracle.

His relationships are now healthier, and his jealous feelings no longer plague him.

The circulation problems he was

experiencing and the burning in the soles of

his feet have cleared as well.

> It's not forgetting that heals.
> It's remembering.
> Amy Greene Bloodroot

Chana Klein

Then There Is the Spirit

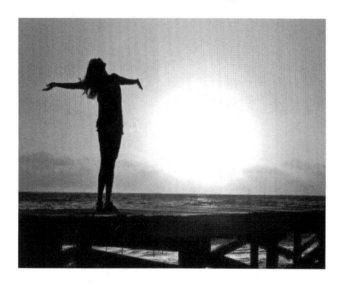

When it's dark, we search for light.
When we hurt, we search for relief.
When the air is bad, we search for fresh air.

Light FROM the Darkness of Illness & Physical Disability

When it's raining, we search for shelter.

When cold, we search for warmth.

When in danger, we search for safety.

Just as being hungry causes our body to
search for food, being ill causes our Spirit to
search for healing.

That is what a human is programmed to do.

That is the natural response.

Each of us is inherently gifted with a
natural response to find what we need.
So naturally when illness strikes, the Spirit
sparks us to find healing.

Chana Klein

Our hurting or suffering triggers that
natural response, which causes us to search,
and to find Light.

Avoiding facing our darkness, only makes it
darker.

Allowing our mind and body to experience
our darkness, facilitates our getting unstuck
from that darkness.

Facing our darkness triggers the activation
of what I believe to be our natural healing
response that I call "The Spirit."

Light FROM the Darkness of Illness
& Physical Disability

The body naturally wants to, and knows
how to, heal itself.

By focusing on our darkness, we cause our
Spirit, in its natural way, to go toward the
Light.

The Spirit animates us to complete our
inner healing work.

Then we find Healing Light.

Chana Klein

An Example in My Life

Several years ago, as part of one of the various training programs that I attended, I was tested on my own sensory integration systems.

According to my results, I have only one out of fourteen sensory integration systems that functions.
That is, kinesthetic.

A year later, at another kind of training, which was on "working memory," I was tested to have no working memory at all.

Light FROM the Darkness of Illness & Physical Disability

My examiners always wonder how I function.

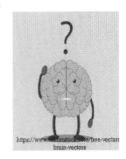

And yet, I function amazingly well, probably better than they do.

Even now, I have recently written five books. This is the second.

I wake up, usually, before 6 am. Every weekday, I write, and then at 8:30 am, I leave for Torah Learning. which often goes until noon, or later if there are additional classes.

Chana Klein

Then, I return home to my work with
clients, successfully healing all kinds of
maladies.

I do more writing between clients and other
activities.
I learn Torah in classes for 3 to 5 hours/day,
a lot of it in Hebrew, and I remember most
of what I learn.

I am trilingual, a licensed Spanish teacher,
and finally, after much struggle, understand
the Hebrew text we study in the shiurim
(classes) that I attend.

So, with a non-functioning brain and a

messed up sensory system how do I

function so well?

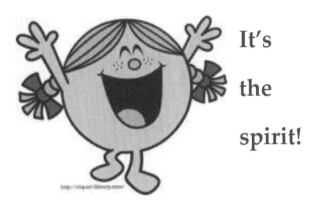

It's

the

spirit!

We may get diagnosis after diagnosis.

But give me a spirit that wants to do a task

and I will show you success, no matter what

the diagnosis.

Chana Klein

In my experience with more ADHD clients than I can count, I find that when a person who has ADHD wants to do a task and has interest in it, there is no ADHD.
That is the Spirit!

When there is suffering, the body and/or mind knows how to heal itself.

The Spirit overcomes it all and gets the job done.
When one suffers, that suffering may find an answer in the body, the mind, and/or the spirit.

When guided by an experienced
practitioner to feel the suffering and process
it, the Spirit heals the person.

How does this happen?

The suffering we feel taps into the
Spirit.

It taps into the human spirit, which has no
limits.

The human spirit defies all physical and
mental diagnoses.

The suffering, when we allow ourselves to feel it, awakens our human spirit to find a solution.
Once the negativity is processed and cleared, the human spirit overcomes and succeeds.

Once cleared of the negative emotions, the spirit finds a way for the mind and body to heal.

Beyond my wildest dreams, I recovered from illnesses that I expected to mess me up, to cripple me, and even to kill me.

For example, when I learned that I had been
suffering from cancer, not wanting to
subject myself to chemo, radiation or any
other medical treatment, I went home to
die.

What got me better?

There is a section on that recovery in this
book.

But at the root all the healing, I believe, is
the Spirit.

Babies, children, teens, adults, we all have
that spark that can face the suffering, the
spark that stops our resisting, that figures
out how we will heal, and does that healing.

"Like Cures Like."

"Dark Cures Dark."

And we become healthy.

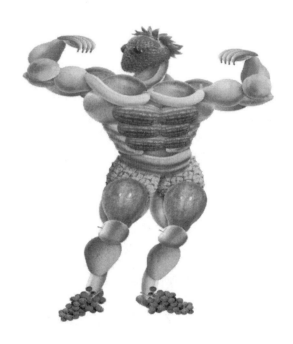

The Torah Sources of "Like Cures Like" & "Dark Cures Dark"

"Light FROM the Darkness Healing" is rooted in very, very old healing principles.

The concepts of "Like Cures Like" and "Dark Cures Dark" are first brought forth in our Torah.

The Torah, was given about 3400 years ago.

That means that the source of the concept of "Like Cures Like" is one of the oldest in the healing world.

There are at least three stories that I can point to in The Torah text that put forth the concept that "Like Cures Like" and Dark Cures Dark:

1. The Israelites are commanded to heal their snake bites by looking at a copper, venomous snake.
2. Moses makes bitter water sweet by using a bitter branch.
3. The way we are commanded to make pots kosher, i.e. to kasher them, is another example of "Like Cures Like."

These are explained in the next pages:

<u>The Harmer that Heals</u>

The story:
The Israelites cried:

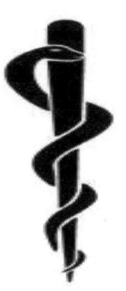

"Why has He (God) brought us up from *Mitzrayim* (Egypt) to die in the desert, for there is no bread and there is no water, and our souls are repulsed with the insubstantial bread?"

The Torah tells us that God's retribution for this complaining was swift.

In no time, the camp was overrun with venomous snakes.

162

Chana Klein

Many Israelites were fatally bitten.

How They Healed:

> "And the people came to Moshe and
> said: 'We have sinned' . . ."
> "And G-d said to Moshe,
> 'Make for yourself a venomous snake and
> place it upon a tall pole, and it shall come
> to pass that anyone who is bitten, let him
> look upon it and he will live.' And Moshe
> made a copper snake . . ."
> (Bamidbar (Numbers) 21:8)

What we are reading in the book of

Bamidbar is that the malady of snake bites

is cured by focusing on a replica of the

venomous snake that bit them.

Looking at the snake, in essence, recreates

the snake-bite experience.

(Dark curing dark.)

Light FROM the Darkness of Illness & Physical Disability

But the person looking at the venomous snake maintains control of the experience while looking.

S/he could stop at any time, unlike during the original snake event when the person had no control.

S/he gets healed of the snake bite by re-experiencing it.

In other words, "Like Cures Like."
"Dark Cures Dark."

Reliving the "dark" experience of the snake bite, cures the snake bite.

Bitter Water Made Sweet by a Bitter Tree

Moses uses a bitter stick of tree wood to sweeten bitter waters.

"Like Cures Like"

From the Book of Shemot (Exodus) Chapter 15:

22. Moses brings Israel out from the Red Sea, and they went into the wilderness of Shur. They went three days in the wilderness and found no water.
23. When they came to Marah, they could not drink the water of Marah because it was bitter; therefore it was named Marah which

24. And the people grumbled against Moses, saying, "What shall we drink?"
25. And he (Moses) cried to the Lord, and the Lord showed him a tree which

165

and he threw it into the water,
and the water became sweet.

The bitter water is made sweet using a bitter
branch.

"Like Cures Like."

Making Unkosher Pots Kosher

The first time I ever heard the concept
of "Like Cures Like" was when I was
making my kitchen kosher.

Rabbi Brodd from Chabad explained to me,

as he was kashering my kitchen in 1994,

that the way a pot became unkosher (traif)

is how it is treated to become kosher.

So, if a pot became unkosher by cooking

bacon, which

is not kosher,

in it, on top

of a fire, then

we restore

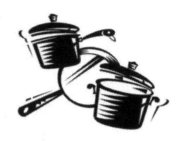

the pot to kosher by heating that pot on top

of a fire.

And if we made the pot traif (unkosher) by

cooking a liquid in it, like a soup that is not

kosher, then we must kasher it with boiling

water, i.e. a liquid.

> **The emotion that can break your
> heart is sometimes the very one
> that heals it . . .
> Nicholas Sparks, At First Sight**

As It Is Absorbed . . .

The basic rule of kashering is *k'bolo kach polto*, a Hebrew expression that means, literally, "as it is absorbed, so is it purged."

In other words, the way a potentially kosher pot became unkosher determines how to make it kosher.

In the same way as it is absorbed, it releases what it has absorbed.

Like Cures Like in Healing

Similarly, for an ill or troubled person, the way s/he became ill, or troubled, would be the pathway to becoming well again.

"Like Cures Like" means that the cure for suffering is to create a similar kind of suffering in the person. So, we have the person re-experience a snapshot of that experience while holding the appropriate acupressure points.

However, the difference here is that the client controls the suffering that s/he creates, unlike the original suffering, which s/he had not been able to control.

In summary, we kasher (make pure) a utensil in the same way it became impure.

And in healing, the way we suffered, or became ill, is the way we cure that suffering, by mentally and/or emotionally repeating it in our mind's eye.

How do we do this today?
We do this by holding the related Chinese Medicine acupressure points to create the flow which encourages the process of healing.

Chana Klein

"We ask patients to re-experience an emotion from past within the context of doing NET.
We're asking them to go back and briefly relive a memory and in reliving that memory they produce a feeling and that feeling is an important "Like Cures Like" component of the NET process.
This extinguishes the conditioned response and the emotions attached to the image."
NET Manual p 109

When I use this technique with my clients,

they report that their symptoms are

alleviated and do not return.

I have had the same results when a

practitioner works the technique on me.

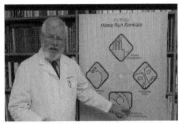 This incredibly effective technique, that was created by Dr. Scott Walker, DC and is managed hands-on by Dr. Deb Walker, DC, is called Neuro Emotional Technique (NET), and has been scientifically validated at Thomas Jefferson University Hospital in Philadelphia.

(For details of those studies go to http://www.netmindbody.com)

More "Like Cures Like" in History

We first heard about "Like Cures Like" from Hippocrates (460-370 BC), the Father of Medicine.

> "By similar things a disease is produced and through the application of the like, is cured."
> Hippocrates (460-370 BC), 'Father of Medicine.

Homeopathy is based on the principle of "Like Cures Like."

According to homeopathic understanding, that which a substance is capable of causing, it is also capable of curing.

173

Light FROM the Darkness of Illness & Physical Disability

In the 16th century, the pioneer of pharmacology, <u>Paracelsus,</u> declared that small doses of "what makes a man ill also cures him."

> *"Paracelsus (German-Swiss physician)"*, *Britannica Online Encyclopedia, Encyclopædia Britannica*, retrieved *2009-03-24*

The term "homeopathy" was coined by Samuel Hahnemann, MD and first appeared in print in 1807.
Hahnemann expanded its meaning and principles in the 19th century.

> Homeopathic medicines are prescribed according to "Like Cures Like." also known as the "Law of Similars."

Dean ME (2001), **Homeopathy and "The Progress of Science** *(PDF), Hist Sci,* **39** *(125 Pt 3): 255–83,* <u>*PMID*</u> <u>*11712570*</u>

Chana Klein

Second only to Hippocrates among the
founders of medicine was another Greek
physician, Galen (130-200 CE), skilled in
anatomy and physiology.
He also wrote of natural cure by the likes.
Galen was recognized as the authority in
medicine for more than 1000 years.

We return now, to summarize our discussion of
Dark Cures Dark, which I derived from the
principle of Like Cures Like.

Our natural response is to want to hide from the
dark.
But that is not the path to healing.

We need to face the dark, feel it to its fullest, and then we heal.

Dark Cures Dark

In summary, when I try to fill my head with positive thoughts that I do not yet really feel, I am being incongruent with myself.

That creates imbalance and conflict in my body.

It is more healing of negative thoughts to really face them as they are, no matter how negative or dark.

Feel those images and thoughts to the fullest.

Then see the light that comes into you. Experience your darkness so that you may experience the Light that you want to feel.

My darkness is cured by re-experiencing the darkness event in a controlled way.

Then I get the Light!

Not Despite . . . But Because

D isability – What Do We Do with It?
Who doesn't have some sort of
disability, either in mind, in body, or even
in spirit?

The question is: What do we do with it?

Does it stop us?

Or, is it the stuff that creates our success?

Do we achieve success despite our disability

. . . or because of it?

Because of My Crutches

I have run a half-mile in 3 ½ minutes on my crutches.

When I did not need crutches to walk, I was never able to travel that fast. It is not despite

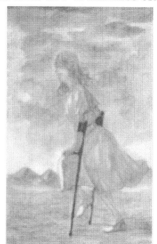

my crutches that I could fly down the street . . . but because of them.

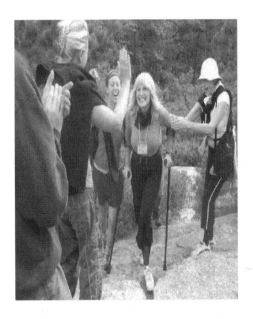

Getting to the top of a 4-mile mountain in 2004.
Only a few of the 70 in the group made it to the top
as I just had. Lucky someone had a camera.

Historical Giants

In studying the lives of leaders like Moses, Jacob, Lincoln, FDR, JFK, and other historical giants, it glares out at me that each of these greats suffered some form of disability that interfered with his life.

Moses

Moses had a speech problem, a great challenge for a national leader. But it was because of that speech difficulty that people believed in Moses as God's prophet.

The people saw that Moses' speech problem

disappeared when he was speaking for

God.

At those times, God would speak through

Moses.

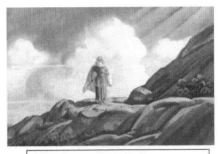

http://www.freebibleimages.org

So, Moses' speech was clear.

This caused the people to believe even more

In Moses as God's prophet.

When God was speaking through Moses they saw that Moses had no speech problem.

Not despite . . . but because of Moses' speech difficulty, were people more aware of Moses as God's prophet!

Jacob

Jacob suffered sciatic nerve pain as a result of a battle with the angel of Eisav, his brother.

Jacob was victorious. (Genesis 32:25)

I imagine the pain Jacob had to live with presented great challenges with all the traveling he had to do, even in getting on and off the wagons on which he rode.

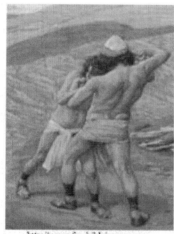

http://www.freebibleimages.org

Jacob traveled all the way down to Egypt with that pain.

After his victory over the angel, Jacob is told, "No longer is your name Jacob, but Israel, for you fought with God and with man and overcame."   Genesis 32:28

184

Chana Klein

A name change is an indication that a person is accessing another part of his soul.

Jacob's pain and his victory were what preceded his name change.

Because of the pain that Jacob acquired in the battle, he got to know, from that time onward, the part of himself that can wrestle with man, and even with God, and can overcome.

Not despite . . . but because of the pain, Jacob endured, he became victorious and became a Beacon of Light for his children and for those after him.

Lincoln

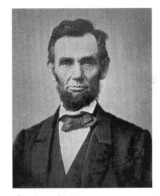

History tells us that Abe Lincoln suffered from severe depression.

"Abraham Lincoln was famously melancholy, experiencing periods of such deep depression throughout his lifetime that he contemplated suicide and spent weeks at a time bedridden."

"http://www.politico.com/magazine/story/2015/10/politics-mental-illness-history-213276#ixzz4I4Xy5CeU

http://tinyurl.com/nbz3aeq)

Yet, history tells us also that Lincoln's office was always open to listening to individuals who requested his help.

His own depression was the thing that made him more compassionate to others. His compassion contributed much to his greatness as president.

> "The opposition researchers of today would   have been very eager to discover Lincoln's propensity for depression," says presidential historian Michael Beschloss.
> "If they had, we might have lost perhaps our greatest president." Ibid

FDR

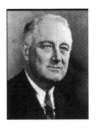

Franklin Delano Roosevelt (FDR) had polio since the age of 39.

His wife, Eleanor, shared that it was his polio that shaped his character as president, and defined his presidency.

> "He had contracted polio in 1921, at age 39, and never recovered the use of his paralyzed legs. Eleanor, his wife, said this experience of struggling and failing to conquer the disease broke him out of the isolation of his background as a patrician who had lived a life of ease and privilege. In his experience with polio, he learned what it was like to struggle, and fail, but to persevere."
>
> FDR: The President Who Made America Into a Superpower - http://tinyurl.com/yay86l3u

JFK

Then there was John Fitzgerald Kennedy (JFK). I personally found his story inspiring and revealing. But not for the usual reasons.

The part that inspired me most is what JFK did with his illness.

For JFK, 50% of his lifetime had been spent in bed, unable to function because of various diagnoses ranging from Addison's Disease to Leukemia.

Light FROM the Darkness of Illness
& Physical Disability

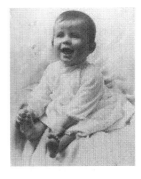

From the time that
JFK was a newborn,
he was ill.

He was given his last
rights at least five
times, the first being just after he was born.
When JFK's older brother, Joe, was born,
their father started calling Joe "President,"
as that was his father's wish for him.

When Jack (JFK, as we know him) was born,
he was already deathly ill.
So, his father's wish for him was simply that
he "live."

Chana Klein

Most of JFK's time, when he attended
Choate Preparatory School in Connecticut,
was spent sick, confined to Choate's
infirmary.

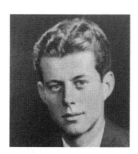 There, it is said, JFK
developed other skills.
He had to develop a
talent for keeping
people interested in
conversing with him, so that he would have
people to talk to while confined to bed.

Light FROM the Darkness of Illness & Physical Disability

While confined to bed, he brought his reading speed up to 1200 words per minute, reading 10 books each week.

He particularly studied "leadership" and had an almost obsessive fascination with politics.

JFK was not an honor student or even a good student.
He graduated from Choate below the middle of his class.

The headmaster even tried to have JFK expelled the night before graduation.

Chana Klein

JFK was a known troublemaker and leader of a group of rabble-rousers that called themselves "The Muckers Club."

Clearly, it was not his great academic *abilities* that got JFK the epitome of worldly success – becoming the 35th President of the United States.

Rather, his *disabilities* created his greatness as President:

I found the following insight by Webster Tarpley, author, historian, journalist, lecturer, that supports my "Not Despite .... But Because" awareness of JFK:

Light FROM the Darkness of Illness & Physical Disability

"Kennedy was brought in originally expected to be a world puppet.

His pro-Nazi father, Joseph P. Kennedy, bootlegger, speculator, would guarantee that Kennedy would be obedient to the establishment. They figured JFK was a sex maniac who could be manipulated through that.

But through his personal suffering, Kennedy had discovered a personal sense of himself that went beyond just being a puppet.

He began to think about things like economic recovery, world peace, having a space program, making deals with the Soviets, cutting the Federal Reserve down to size, and a whole series of other things like real civil rights reform. He began pulling troops out of Vietnam as well."

It was his personal illness that made Kennedy the greatest, most sincere, and trustworthy of all presidents.

From this commentary, we can conclude that had Kennedy not had his illnesses and disabilities, he probably would not have reached the level of greatness that he did.

Rather, it was his *disabilities*, the disabilities that forced him to stay in bed, during which he created and accessed his own inner gifts.
It was not despite Kennedy's disabilities . . . but because of them that JFK developed such incredible greatness.

People on the Spectrum

A lot of my work is with people on the Autism Spectrum.

My experience with these beautiful souls leads me to believe that many of them have achieved greatness, or can achieve that greatness, not despite . . . but because of their Autism Spectrum Disorder.

There are those in history who are believed to have had Asperger's, which is on the Autism Spectrum.

Each had many of the characteristics of that syndrome, like a lack of ability to recognize social cues, avoidance of eye contact, a tendency to rock back and forth, coupled with an obsession with, and intense focus on, certain subject matter.

Historical giants such as Marie Curie,

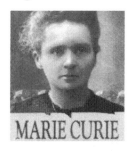

Light FROM the Darkness of Illness & Physical Disability

Albert Einstein,

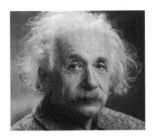

Mozart,

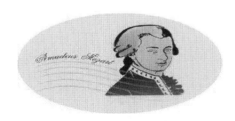

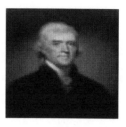

Thomas Jefferson,

are thought to have had Asperger's.

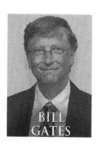

Recently added to that list

is Bill Gates.

Is it despite their

Asperger's traits . . . or because of those

traits that each became so successful?

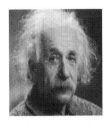 Did Einstein do his
brilliant work of focusing
on small details for hours
and coming to creative
conclusions despite his Asperger's trait of
intense focus on subject matter . . . or
because of it?

Did Van Gogh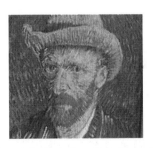
add beautiful
color and abstract
edges to his
paintings despite the seizures he developed
while in the hospital . . . or because of those
seizures?

Chana Klein

How many of our disabilities are the material out of which our success is created?

Do we do great things despite disability . . . or because of it?

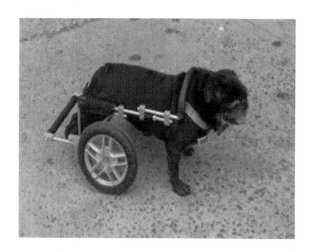

My Own Story:

"You have Reflex Sympathetic Dystrophy (RSD, aka CRPS) and you are not returning to work," the orthopedic surgeon announced to me.

I had not planned on ever ending my teaching career.

I had believed that retirement would happen for me after my soul leaves this world, and even then, I used to tell people, that Heaven, for me, will be a classroom filled with kids.

Chana Klein

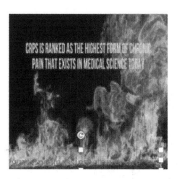

The pain of the disease with which I was diagnosed is described by victims of this illness as having one's veins filled with lighter fluid and then lighting a match. That is what it was like for me, as well.

I traveled hundreds of miles to be treated by the RSD medical doctor who was considered the world's guru of the disease.

He diagnosed me with full body RSD and
predicted, with certainty, that within a year,
I would be confined to a wheelchair.

What CAN I Do?

I was not able to dress myself without
assistance, and had already lost my
ability to walk.
As I lay on my back with two pillows under
my knees, I asked myself:
"What CAN I do?"

"I can learn!" was the answer that quickly
came to me.

Whereas I had been learning Torah intensively for more than 21 years, I, now, had to take some of that time that had been spent on Torah and use it to learn to heal myself.

I enrolled in Alternative Medicine courses and trainings, which eventually led to many alternative practitioner certifications.

Eventually, I completed training in more than 20 different healing modalities of Alternative Medicine Certifications.

I found out about coaching as a profession from one of the Alternative Medicine students and signed up for the first of many years of those trainings the next day.

Within a few years, I was certified in many schools of coaching, in addition to many mind-body modalities.

Using what I was learning, my physical condition got better and better.

The pain dissipated and my ability to function increased and continues to do that each day.
In 2016, I regained my ability to walk.

Chana Klein

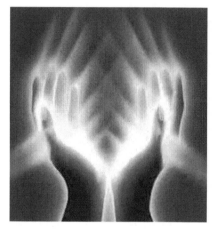

I know that I never would have gotten the endless trainings and certifications, nor would I have been able to help the people who became my clients, had I not been so disabled that I was forced to leave what I was doing, really, to leave what, at the time, I loved doing.

How could I have known that I would be able to grow my brain and my body in such

different, expansive ways, to be who I am
today, to do what I do, not despite . . . but
because of my disability?

To Shape Our Souls

Does God give us these disabilities to
shape our souls?

Are these the things that force us to reach
above, and then reach deep inside, to enable
our inner greatness to emerge?

I look at my disabilities, of which I have
many, both in mind and body.

Chana Klein

I see them as the source of my very
meaningful life.

I see them as the root of my being able to be
there in just the right way for another
person.

I see my disabilities as giving me additional
insight into understanding a drop of how
the world works, and of understanding
what inspires another to go on to experience
victory over others, and even more
importantly, over oneself.

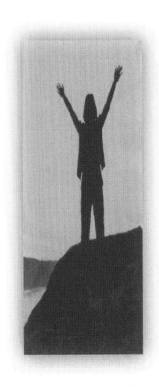

Not despite the
challenges
brought before us
. . . but because of
those challenges,
do
we find the inner
greatness within
ourselves, and
the ability to
express that
greatness.

Not despite . . . but because of our
disability, are we able to achieve what we
do.

Chana Klein

The Power in the Search:
Where Do We Find the Cure?
(For Parents and Loved Ones)

Hopeless Situations

We experience so many life situations. Sometimes we lose hope, which makes things feel so much worse.

But then there are those times when all hope feels nonexistent and an answer, a solution, somehow appears from an

unexpected place.

What is that?

How do we access it?

To a person in search of work,

or in search of a partner,

or an answer to a health issue . . .

From where does the answer come?

Could it be that the answer is right in front

of us?

Yet, we are not able see it?

How often is it that we actually do find an answer?

How many times does the problem seem to just go away, once we make the effort to search for an answer?

Could it be the effort of that search that brings us to the solution?

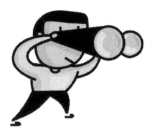

In our Torah

Hagar

In our Torah, Hagar, the mother of Yishmael, was expelled from Avraham's house.
She was left on her own with her baby.

The water that Avraham had given her for the journey was used up.

I can't imagine the pain she experienced that made her, as his mother, say:

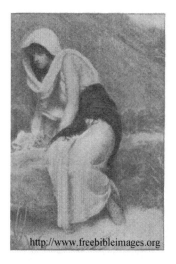

Chana Klein

"Let me not see the death of the child."

(Genesis 21:16)

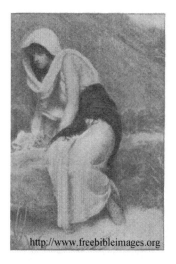

http://www.freebibleimages.org

Then she left him to sit in another place, a place where she would not be with her son to witness his death.

But was there really no water?

Our Torah tells us:

"Then, God opened her (Hagar's) eyes and
she perceived a well of water."
(Genesis 21:19)

But the text tells us that the water that
Hagar saw had not been created by God just
at that moment, just for her.

God merely opened Hagar's eyes to see
what had already been there.
Really, it was there the whole time.

Perhaps so many of our answers are there
the whole time.
We just don't see them right away.

Yosef

"The brothers of Yosef," as they are called in Genesis 42:3, search for Yosef in every part of the city.

The brothers regretted having sold Yosef into slavery. Now they were determined to find him, redeem him, and bring him back to Yakov. (Rashi Genesis 42:3)

Their father, Yakov, had instructed them to go directly to the center market.

But in their search for Yosef, they wandered through the city exploring side streets and alleys, markets, stores, inns, and theaters.

Unbeknownst to the brothers, Yosef was now the Viceroy of Egypt.

Yosef's security guards saw the brothers' suspicious behavior and reported it directly to Yosef.

They were brought before him (for questioning.)

There they were, standing before the object of their search.

Yet, they did not know that they had found him.

They did not know that the one questioning them was their brother, Yosef.

> "Joseph recognized his brothers, but they did not recognize him."
> Genesis 42:8

How many times have we found what we are in search of, and still had no idea that it was right in front of us?

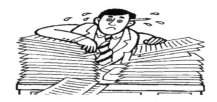

The Search for Rory

(Recreated from a story I heard.)

It was a time of war between the people

who lived in the flatlands of the desert and

the people who lived high up on Mount

Ramon, the highest mountain in Southern

Israel.

It was a dark night when the people of the

mountain raided the people of the desert.

They pillaged through homes.

They climbed into the bedroom window of

Rory, waking him up.

Chana Klein

They grabbed him and carried him away.

Rory was on the Autistic Spectrum.

He was his mom's only child.

By two-and-a-half-years-old, Rory had lost

his speech ability.

Food for Rory, had to be a certain texture,

color and place on the plate, for him to eat

it.

He avoided physical touch.

But he was attached to his cushy, stuffed

alligator toy.

Light FROM the Darkness of Illness & Physical Disability

Rory's screams pierced his mom's ears with
the quick shuffling sound of intruders.
Slamming the door open against the wall,
his mom flew into his room.

His toy alligator lay in his bed . . . alone.
She was frantic.
"He can't express himself.
He won't know where he is.
What will they do to him?
How will he eat?"

She dialed the phone number for the Police.
They showed up quickly.
They searched the area.

There were no mountain people in sight. The mountain men got away and were likely headed up the mountain.

"Oh, dear God, please, please, please, make them find my baby," the mom prayed.

The police set out to make their way up the pathway that the mountain people must have taken the child.

But the police were not mountain people and were not experienced in searching the trails in the mountain or in climbing it.

223

Yet, they assisted each other over rocks,

pushing their way through undergrowth on

the ground.

It was not working.

They looked for another path and embarked

up that one.

They kept trying.

After hours of effort, it was daybreak.

After more hours, the sun set, and rose

again.

And then it was night again.

The rugged mountain proved to be a huge

undertaking.

Chana Klein

They feared they were going to lose their
men.

They were only 200 feet up the 3,402-foot-
high mountain.
The senior officer could not foresee that
they would ever be able to reach where the
mountaineers had brought the child.

The police called on the army for assistance.
The soldiers arrived and they, too,
attempted to climb the mountain to where
the toddler was likely being held.

The army people knew a little bit more than
the police knew about getting up the
mountain.

With picks and huge iron rods they
attempted to make the climb.

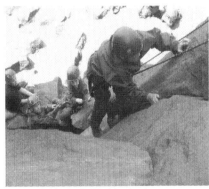 They
held each
other up
with
ropes.

activities/rock-climbing.html

Yet, it was appearing to be impossible to
travel very far on the treacherous terrain.

Night came and daybreak, and then another
day and another.

The men were exhausted.

They had succeeded in climbing only 400
feet.

At this rate, they will not be able to get to
the child.

This was proving to be an impossible
mission.

Dejected and powerless, they felt terrible.

They prepared to pack their gear to head
back down.

As they packed, several of the men looked up in the distance at the challenging topography.

There, they saw the mom descending. "Look! It's the mom. How did she do that???"

The mom was coming down the huge mountain.

Chana Klein

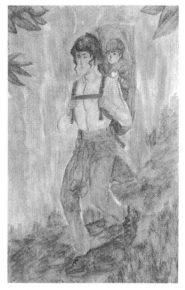

She had a toddler strapped to her back, who was holding a toy alligator tightly to his chest.

This mom was coming down the treacherous mountain that the men were not able to fathom how to climb.

Three of the men climbed up to where the mom was trekking, in order to assist her.

She stood in front of them on the landing.
"How did you get up there? We, the protective forces, are the most skilled in the country.
And we were not able to go higher than 400 feet.
How did you get to the top?
How did you get the child?"

She looked at the group and explained with the simplest and clearest explanation:

"It's not your child!"

The Lesson

What we learn from this story about finding a cure:
This story takes place in Southern Israel.
But it could be anywhere . . . anywhere that a parent or anyone else searches for answers.

The power of a parent's search, the power of that love and determination to find what is missing.

The power of a parent to do for a child what no one else is capable of.

Light FROM the Darkness of Illness & Physical Disability

I have worked with many parents in their search for healing, in search of answers to their child's issue.

I find it amazing how a child, whose mother, father, or one who cares so deeply, searches in all places for his healing, somehow gets healed.

I often wonder if it is the search itself that offers the solution.

My Story

My son was very ill, in and out of consciousness.

It began at birth, with his difficulty breathing, and within months, a seizure disorder.

One illness led to another and another. We were told he would not be with us much longer.

Light FROM the Darkness of Illness
& Physical Disability

I screamed, silently, each day, and each
night, from the agony of each additional
diagnosis, from the parental torment of the
illness, and more from the fear of losing
him.

At the same time, I had to look ahead.
I foresaw that if, someday, after he leaves
this world, if I find that a real cure exists,
and I had not accessed it, I would feel
unbearable regret and guilt.

According to the doctors, there was no
hope.
His blood levels were slipping, and his
consciousness did not exist.

It was only a matter of time.

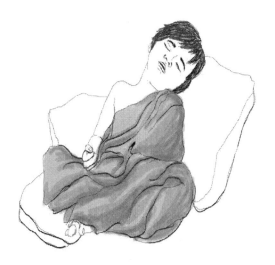

He was holding on.

And I was holding on to him.

I decided to not leave any avenue
unsearched, even though I had no hope of
finding an answer.

In those days, before the Internet, I
managed to extend my search as far as
Europe.
I felt I needed to be at peace with the surety
that once the inevitable occurred, that I had
tried everything and searched everywhere
possible.

Did I find an answer? No!
Did I find a solution to the orchestra of
sounds and gasps he made when breathing?
to his non-stop seizures? No!

Chana Klein

to his almost non-existent platelet count?

to countless abnormal blood levels?

to his toxic liver?

brain tumor?

brain aneurysm?

internal bleeding?

subglottal laryngeal stenosis?

subglottal tumors?

loss of speech?

hallucinations causing an inability to eat

because of the moving worms he saw in his

food?

abdominal pain?

urethral pain?

test after test?

extended periods of unconsciousness?

surgeries, hospitalizations, medications?

Did I find answers to these medical

problems?

No! I did not.

Not a one.

Did my son recover?

Did he improve?

Did he get any better with all that I did as a

mother searching for a cure for my darling

baby, for the child that I loved so very

much?

At ten-years-old, he began to show some

life.

Chana Klein

His father remarked to me at the time, that
our son has not had a seizure in three
months.

His other levels were so dangerously out-of-
whack.
He still seemed so sick, that I had not
realized that something did get better.

And then slowly, his ferritin level went up.
The platelets recovered.
His pain lessened.
He was breathing more freely.

Eventually, he was no longer slipping in
and out of consciousness.

After age ten and a half, he never again had
another seizure.

Dr. Stanley Resor, the head of the Seizure
Clinic of Colombia Presbyterian Hospital
told us that no medication can offer 100%
seizure control. (80% control is the best that
a medication can offer.)

"It, therefore, must be that his seizures are
less because *he* is better," the doctor
claimed.

Now, when I waited outside his Hebrew
School classroom for the next episode of his
passing out, there was nothing to wait for.

He came out of class on time, and I no longer had to carry him to the car.

And slowly, beyond my hopes, and beyond what I ever thought could be, he got better, really better, until he eventually was 100% healthy, to this day, thank You, God.

All along, I thought it was medical answers that I was trying to find.

But there never were any real medical remedies to point to.

As his mother, I had searched for a way to make my child heal from all the maladies

that affected his darling, hurting brain and
body.

We never found a medical cure.
We never found a tangible remedy.

But we did find healing, total and complete
healing.

I did not understand, at the time, that the
answers might have been there all along.
But to reveal those answers, I had to look
for them.
I had to search.

Chana Klein

From the place where we keep on trying,
from the place where we don't give up,
that is where the answers show up,
and that is from where the problems and
maladies seem to disappear.

The Almighty sees our effort, and then He
reveals the answers that were there all
along.

Hagar, in the only way she knew, searched
for water for her child.

The brothers of Yosef did the best they
could to amend their mistake and find their
brother, whom they had at first left in the

pit, and later sold him as a slave to the
Yishmaelites.

Rory's mom, who was determined to find
her child and get him home . . .
And my own search for a cure for my child.

All those searches did not result in any new
findings.
In each case, the answers were revealed just
with the effort to find them.

> "I shall raise my eyes to the
> mountains, from where will my help
> come? My help is from the Lord, the
> Maker of Heaven and earth." (Psalm
> 121)

The answers are already here.

The Master of the Universe opens our eyes commensurate with our effort.

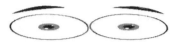

The Almighty reveals the light to those who search the darkness.

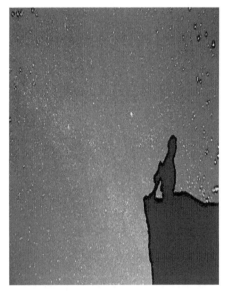

That is the Light FROM the Darkness.

Resistance & Illness

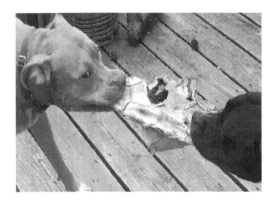

What we resist, persists.

The more I hold onto the object to get it away from Nala, the pit bull, the stronger that Nala holds onto it, keeping me from having it.

246

So, it is with illness.

The stronger I try to fight my illness, the

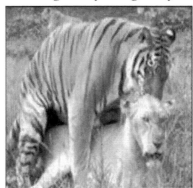

more it engulfs me. This lion is resisting the grasp of the tiger, causing the tiger to hold on more tightly. https://wn.com/lion_vs_tiger_fight_videos

Fighting your illness is really fighting your own body.

Embracing Illness

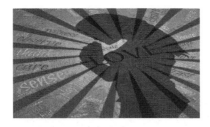

We can't fight disease.

We must embrace it . . .

and thank it for its deep lessons.

"You can't get to where you want until you are okay being where you are." (Dr. Scott Walker, DC, Creator of NET)

Chana Klein

Clearing Cancer

Preface to My Remarks on Cancer

I want to preface my remarks with acknowledgement for those who have been helped in some way by Western Medicine.

Western Medicine has its time and place, and its strengths and weaknesses.

Light FROM the Darkness of Illness & Physical Disability

It may be a good system in a critical emergency, and for complicated surgical procedures and traumas.

If I break a bone or have a problem with my eyes, I go to a Western Medicine physician. I have a great Ophthalmologist, Dr. Joseph Fishkin, MD, who has done a great job with my eyes and a wonderful Orthopedist, Dr. Raphael Levine, MD, who always steers me away from anything invasive in treating my legs, and he is always right.

For anything chronic, most physicians insist on one or more medications, or surgery. From all my trainings and experience, I

know that there are so many better
alternatives.

I acknowledge those who have had cancer
and received help from Western Medicine.
However, the success rate according to an
online study (http://tinyurl.com/y95r9egn
telling the 5-year survival rate as its
measure - is that only 2.1% are still alive
five years after chemo.

Not considered or mentioned in the study
was the quality of life of the survivors
during and after the years of receiving
chemo.

I searched the Internet for reports of good
experiences with Chemo and cannot find
any.

I remain open to listening for good news on
that.

I also searched for the success of other
cancer treatments like immunotherapy,
hormone therapy, and radiation.

The horrendous side effects requiring yet
further treatment, and the secondary
cancers caused by these treatments that
could show up years later, would still
convince me to go the way I did.

I had zero side effects and recovered totally.

For those who did get better with Western Medicine, may you continue in good health with increased satisfaction with life.

What I know and write about in this book is my own experience and views, and is based on extensive research.

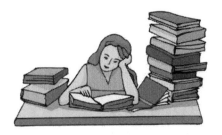

Fighting Cancer

I have heard people say they will "fight" their cancer.

I have heard medical institutions brag about "fighting" cancer.

In that vein, I have also heard people say they will make that Autistic child behave.

I have heard people say they will control whatever . . .

Chana Klein

Issues that we don't want in our person and
in our lives, bring out the fight in us.
But when is that fight not helpful?

How often do we end up realizing that the
thing we are fighting is ourselves?

And even more often, it is ourselves whom
we end up defeating.

We must ask ourselves, is all this resistance
effective?

Can we clear a problem by offering a strong
resistance?

For example, can I get my brain working

better by *resisting* the brain fog that I get

from my ADHD?

Or does "resisting" brain fog bring on even

more brain fog?

And finally,
Can I fight my cancer and win?

The truth is that what we resist persists.

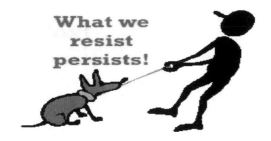

Chana Klein

What The Torah Shows Us About Resisting

We learn the futility of Resistance first, in The Torah, the source of the vastest and greatest wisdom.

In the book of Exodus, we read about the plague of frogs.

God tells Moses:

> "Come to Paraoh and say to him,
> 'So said Hashem (God):
> Send out My people that they may serve
> Me. But if you refuse to send out, behold, I
> shall strike your entire boundary with frogs.
> The River shall swarm with frogs, and they
> shall ascend and come into your palace and
> your bedroom, and your bed, and into the

house of your servants and of your people,
and into your ovens and into your kneading
bowls. And into you and your people and all
your servants will the frogs ascend.' "
Exodus 7:26-29

Does this sound awful or what?

What would you do if you had been there

with frogs in your every living space?

Would you try to kill the frogs?

Would you fight them?

What if there were only one frog?
(or one tumor?)

Chana Klein

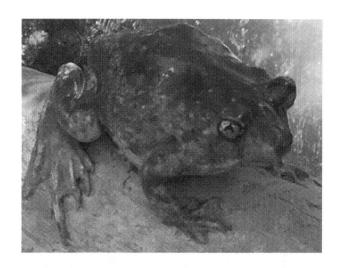

One Gigantic Frog

The plague of frogs in Egypt began with one gigantic frog.

How much damage would you think that one frog could do to a whole people?

What made it possible for that frog to be so powerful?

Rashi says "There was one frog, and when they would hit it, it would spew out bands and bands of little frogs."
(Rashi on Exodus 8:2; Midrash Tanchuma, Shemos, chapter 14; Talmud, Tractate Sanhedrin 67b)

What happened?

God caused one gigantic frog to emerge from the Nile.
When the terrified Egyptians hit the frog, it spewed out smaller frogs.

The more they struck the one frog, the more frogs would come out.

The more frogs came out, the more they would strike them.

Chana Klein

Doesn't this sound like what we do with various challenges, like cancer, like misbehaving children? like brain fog??

We fight it.

We hit it.

We go to destroy it, or him, or her, or them.

And in the process, we destroy ourselves.

The frog was the darkness.

The Egyptians resisted the frog.

The more they resisted, the bigger and more numerous the frogs became.

Eventually, the entire land of Egypt (except for the Jewish region of Goshen) was covered with frogs.

The more they resisted, the worse the situation became.

We can't resist the darkness.

When we try, it only gets darker.

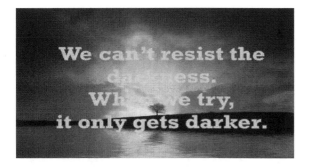

So, what to do when things get awful?

We need to be with it.

Face it.

Feel it.

Grow in it.

My Story

I was so weak.

I couldn't keep my head up.

I wasn't able to eat, or to talk, or to function.

I'd already had a low-grade fever for more

than two years.

Light FROM the Darkness of Illness
& Physical Disability

Because my fever was under 101 degrees,

Dr. Bennett of Beth Israel Hospital insisted

that it was not fever.

But my body felt like it was burning and

anyone who touched me was alarmed by

the heat my body was giving off.

I was also "fighting" anemia with the

medication that Dr. Bennett prescribed for

me.

I was losing that fight.

(Cancer causes anemia and low-grade fever.

I did not know that at the time.)

<u>"I am dying."</u>

Chana Klein

I was scheduled to be a speaker at a local science conference one Shabbos.

Feeling a little better after taking an antibiotic for two days, that had been prescribed by Dr. Bennet, my ex went with me to the conference.

But by Saturday I was feeling sick again. Feeling even worse, as I was presenting to the group, I had to stop speaking for a few moments, as I felt the blood leaving my head.

Light FROM the Darkness of Illness
& Physical Disability

Losing awareness of it being Shabbos, I
asked for someone to raise the air
conditioning, rather than telling anyone that
I was about to pass out.
I didn't want to distract the audience from
the stories I was telling.

You know, we all have our priorities!
I was more concerned about continuing my
presentation, than with the fact that they
may have to carry me out, if I did continue.

So, I grounded myself as I learned to do in
EEM, and was then able to hold myself up.
I then completed my storytelling, grateful
that the audience loved it.

Chana Klein

After my presentation, I asked Dr. Bennett, who was also attending the conference, for a medical visit with him in the hotel lobby.

I had already been complaining to him for more than two years. about not feeling well

That afternoon in the lobby:

"I'm dying," I told him.

"We are all dying," he responded.

"No, I'm dying this week," I said.

"I can look at you and see that you are not sick," was his reply.

"I feel dizzy, like the blood is leaving my head," I continued trying to convince him that I need

help.

"Get Antivert!" he told me,

Then, he offered to send me to Dr. Salant, in

NYC.

That Monday morning, while I was waiting

in Dr. Salant's office, my head rested in my

lap, for I was too weak to hold it up.

Dr. Salant sent me for a CAT Scan.

The Scan identified an intestinal tumor.

He then sent me to Dr. Ferstenberg, a GI

specialist in NYC.

Chana Klein

My first appointment with Dr. Ferstenberg was Wednesday.

Blood studies revealed that I lost four units of blood between Monday and Wednesday.

On my second visit to Dr. Ferstenberg, my ex-husband waited with me in the waiting room for one of the diagnostic tests that Dr. Ferstenberg was about to do.

As I waited, I became freezing cold.

Later, my ex told me that I became very pale and then I lost consciousness.

Light FROM the Darkness of Illness & Physical Disability

My ex, who is a physician and a healer, told me I lost my vitals and was totally unresponsive, no pulse, no breath, etc.

He brought me back by holding certain acupuncture points as we had learned in EEM trainings.

When I saw Dr. Ferstenberg, he told me that my blood was in hemolysis, whatever that meant.

Diagnosis

Eventually, after a CAT scan, a PET scan, and blood studies, several oncologists informed me that I had cancer.

The PET scan and blood studies located the Ovarian cancer as well as the GI tumor.

The diagnosis did not scare me or shock me because I had already felt so very ill and weak for almost 3 years.

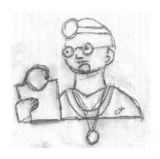

I knew something was terribly wrong and
felt as if I were dying, as I had already told
Dr. Bennett.

My hemoglobin went down to 6. (Normal is
12.9 to 15.9).

So right after seeing Dr. Ferstenberg, Dr.
Bennet, who had told me I am not sick a few
days before, informed me that there is a bed
for me in Beth Israel Hospital and that I am
to have transfusions of several units of
blood that afternoon.

The day after leaving Beth Israel Hospital, I
had a workup in the John Theurer Cancer

Center in Hackensack University Medical
Center.

I was seen by several oncologists.

I listened carefully to their message and
their words.

They
found
tumors in
my small
intestine
and in my ovaries.

Chemo

When I got home, I looked up each chemo drug that they would offer.

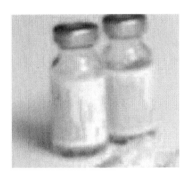

Each drug had the same side effect. Each chemo drug would cause Leukemia within five years of taking it, no matter what kind of cancer the chemo was treating.

Chana Klein

The Oncologists I saw had not shared this
with me.

Rather, I found the information on the
Internet as I looked up each individual
chemo drug.

I was already so weak and sick that I felt
like even one dose of chemo would kill me.

The way the doctors treat a cancer, I just
knew, would kill me right away.
My immune system was not strong enough
to handle even an aspirin, no less a dose of
toxic chemo.

Standard of Care

D octors go by what is called the "Standard of Care."

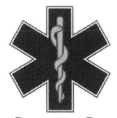

Standard of Care

It is what they are trained in, and they don't know, or want to know, other ways to treat Cancer, or any other illness.

"Standard of Care" means they all do the same thing. That is the "Standard."

If they deviate from this "Standard of Care," they risk being brought up on charges by the medical establishment, with possible loss of their license to practice medicine.

The two leading, known causes of cancer are radiation and chemical toxicity.

Yet, the Standard of Care for cancer is exactly that - Radiation and Chemical Toxicity.

If a patient is harmed by, or dies from, the treatment, as long as the standard of care is followed, the doctor is held blameless.

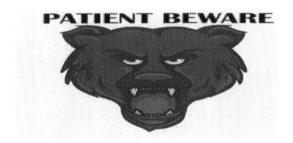

Medical School

The doctor who goes outside the standard of care and actually helps his patients heal, risks public disgrace and loss of his medical license, along with being

brought up on charges by the FDA.

The first Medical Schools were funded by

the pharmaceutical industry.

The model of treating all illness with drugs

remains in place to this day.

Doctors, when attending medical school,

learn primarily, diagnosis and medication.

So that is primarily what they offer.

Basically, they are attempting to treat just

the symptoms of the disease.

The medical schools do not address the root cause of any common illness, often blaming the genetics of the patient.

American Cancer Society

In 2009 after my diagnosis, I looked to the American Cancer Society to see if they could help.

I came upon an article saying that in May of 2013, the American Cancer Society will have its 100th birthday.

Does that mean, I wondered, that after almost 100 years, people have done huge things in science, technology and everything else in the world, but despite the creation of this complicated, conglomerate organization, have not touched on a cure for so many types of cancer, especially after all the time they have existed?

As a healer, I saw that often when there is a huge "benefit to an illness" (see my story on this,) the client is prevented from getting better by their own conscious or subconscious thought.

Does the same apply here?

Is there is a benefit of the illness in the
business of cancer?

The American Cancer Society earns oodles
of money, employs herds of people, has lots
of buildings, etc.

Do they really want to find a cure and give
up all those billions of dollars?
All those buildings?
All those jobs?
All that prestige?

Jailed and Kicked Out

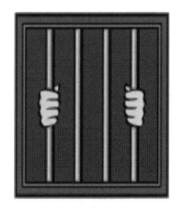

If they do want to find a cure, why did the medical establishment put Dr. Stanislaw Burzynski, MD of the Burzynski Clinic, Harry Hoxsey, Dr. Tullio Simoncini, MD from Italy, and so many others, who had real cures for cancer, in jail?

Light FROM the Darkness of Illness & Physical Disability

Why did they kick them out of the country?
Why did the establishment work so hard at
hiding the successful results of those
professionals?

These doctors and others each found a cure,
a natural cure, that was not costly.

But because they were kicked out by the
establishment, most of them today are in
Mexico and other places where they
presently continue to cure cancer with the
techniques these doctors have created, but
to which we do not have access unless we
leave the country.

Chana Klein

My Take on Cancer: Hindsight of a Recovered Cancer Survivor

I had already been a mind-body practitioner for many years.
I could usually figure out the origin of my clients' issues and figure out how to clear what is ailing them.

Here, I was the client.
Even though I did not have the life-energy needed to do anything, I had to figure this out.

What Created My Cancer?

"Fighting" the cancer, which my body created, and invited to reside in my body, is really fighting my own body.

My body created the cancer.
My body created the cancer as a way to absorb and to localize what could have occurred throughout my whole body.

It was like the first tumor was taking the rap for the rest of my body.
I believe the cancer was my body's way of dealing with my negative emotions.

Chana Klein

It was my body's way of localizing, into one spot, the shock and the bad feelings that had been plaguing me.

The cancer took on all the harmful energy that could have easily affected my whole body.
In my body's effort to save me, the occurrence of the cancer, was localized into one tumor, rather than into my whole body.

In other words, all that negative energy became localized into a cancerous tumor.

The cancer that my body created was my body's way of trying to help me to survive.

Light FROM the Darkness of Illness & Physical Disability

Localizing my shock and other painful emotions into one place (the cancer), likely saved the rest of my body.

I had to look at what created my cancer. The cancer was created by my body to solve a problem that I had not addressed myself.

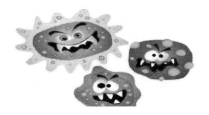

Chana Klein

Natural Detox

My illness forced me to begin to detox
my body and my life.

Another Light FROM the Darkness!

I lost my appetite.

I was unable to speak more than two words

together without passing out.

It was as if God was giving me these

symptoms, forcing me to let go of

everything, including foods that were not good for me, including thoughtless words that could be harmful at times, and toxic substances that had been filling my body and my house.

Clearing cancer meant letting go of relationships, foods, mold and other allergens, and of utmost importance, toxic emotions.

A big part of getting stricken with cancer involves experiencing a shock, plus being exposed to an environmental toxin of some sort.

Chana Klein

Anything that depletes the immune system
feeds a cancer.

I hired a company to clear my house of
mold.
Just before my diagnosis, I became aware of
mold as a carcinogen through my search on
the internet for the cause of fever of
unknown origin (FUO.)

After three years of this fever, the Internet
told me it had to be the mold.

I had a mold company discard almost all
my belongings, except of course my clothes.
(There are limits to what a girl will do! Lol)

Toxic Emotions

In years of working with ailments like cancer, I have found that when a client tells me what part of the body is inflicted with cancer, I can tell them which toxic emotion likely initiated it.

Almost all illness begins with a stress, usually a stressful emotion.

Each emotion is connected to a different organ.

For example, lung cancer involves grief.

Liver cancer involves anger.

Chana Klein

Gall bladder cancer involves resentment.
I have found in my practice that breast
cancer is usually a resentment of nurturing
others, etc.

I had to figure out which toxic emotions
caused my Ovarian condition that spread to
my Small Intestine.

Small Intestine involves negative emotions
such as abandonment, vulnerability or
feelings of being lost.

I imagine that the effect of years of
experiencing those negative emotions got
stuck in my body and created a cancer.

Clearing Cancer

Cancer does not spring up overnight. It accumulates in the body for years before it lets us know it is there.

We can clear it though.

It is never too late.

I had to be cleared.

Being a Master Certified Practitioner in Neuro Emotional Technique (NETmindbody.com), I did the technique on myself as well as getting other practitioners to work on me when one was in my area.

I did the same with Eden Energy Medicine (EEM), in which I am a Certified Advanced Practitioner.

EEM has been invaluable in creating flow and balance in my body.

Based on the techniques I learned in EEM, I created other techniques for each issue that arose from of this condition.

Another invaluable tool in working with Cancer is Interactive Guided Imagery, in which I am certified by the Academy for Guided Imagery (AGI).

Interactive Guided Imagery was a must in knowing where the cancer in my body was holding, and in getting it where I wanted it to be.

I did this through visualization of what I imagined the cancer looked like, and of what I imagined my body's natural defenses and processes to be, as they were eliminating my cancer.

Chana Klein

For someone treated by chemo, s/he might
picture the chemo working at eliminating
the cancer.

I have my clients draw what they image in
their mind's eye, which gives them and me
an idea of what the cancer and the
treatment are doing within them at the time.

That gives us a place to begin imaging the
healing.
The power of Imagery as a healing tool is
well documented.

My Decision

I decided to decline the chemo and the radiation that the doctors were pushing.

I explained to the oncologist that I do not want to wonder (while being treated with chemo) whether it is my body being so ill, or if it were a reaction to the poisons in the chemo.

I felt that I needed to deal with this illness in my body without adding the effects of the drugs that they wanted me to receive as the Standard of Care.

Chana Klein

I didn't fight with them.

I just stated my feelings.

I told them what I wanted and what I did
not want.

No one argued with me.

Then, I went home to die.

I figured that at least I may die with dignity
and without the devastating side effects of
the chemo.

I figured that if I were to die, it would be of
my own body's illness rather than the
medical treatment that "fights" a cancer
with poisons and radiation.

While home, I was not well enough to do any chores.

I got around on my hands and knees, for I had to keep my head down in order to 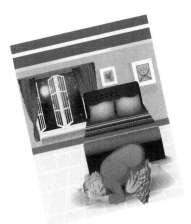 prevent the blood from leaving my head, which in turn would cause me to pass out.

Speaking also caused me to feel like the blood was leaving my head and thereby, passing out.

So, I had to save my words and be
extremely succinct.

I worked purposefully at getting my affairs
in order.

I threw out and deleted anything that might
hurt the feelings of my now ex-husband.

I figured, let him remember our marriage as
happy.
Why should he know my unhappiness?

Let him have just happy memories and feel
good about himself, I mused.

I was greatly comforted knowing he would give me a Jewish burial and say the Mourner's Kaddish for me, which is a Jewish prayer sanctifying God's name after a death.

Having already lost my vitals three times that month, plus after having had a visit to the next world, I was resigned to dying.

My youngest son, Brett, knowing the situation, kept visiting and spending time with me each day.

Getting Better

B ut as time went on, I felt stronger.
I started to realize that I am no longer
feeling like each breath is my last.
I am no longer dying, I realized.

Appetite

I had no appetite.
I believe that the loss of appetite is Heaven's
way of healing us when we are ill enough to
not be able to eat.

Digesting food takes away from the body's energy to heal.

I experienced how illness removes our appetite, leaving us with the energy for the body's inherent healing power to work unencumbered by the digestive process.

After some months, my appetite did return, partially.

I went to an integrative nutritionist and set out to learn, finally, how to eat to be healthy.

Chana Klein

I learned how it is not what I eat that is
important, but rather what I don't eat that
makes me healthy.

Today, still . . . I do not, ever, eat gluten,
cow's milk products, processed sugar,
alcohol, canola and other toxic oils,
carbonated drinks, or soy.

I don't eat anything that has more than one
ingredient when I buy it.
I don't eat anything processed.
I don't eat anything that comes in a package
or in a metal can.

In my mind, the thought of my food having
sat in a metal can for either months and
often years meant that the metal material of
that can, had to be absorbed by the food.
This was not at all healthy for my body.

So, I went through
the house and
discarded every can I
could find, never
again to bring any
can into my house.

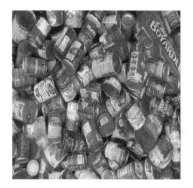

WHAT TO AVOID

After much research, energy testing, and experience with how my clients and I get affected by what we put in our mouth and on our body, I put this list together for them and now for you.

I hope it helps to bring you to Real Healing.

What You Need to Know for Healthy Living

The important focus for healthy eating is not what *to* eat but rather what *NOT* to eat.

Foods to avoid: sugar, gluten - all wheat products including rye, spelt, & barley, pasta, soy, GMO (Genetically Modified Organism) Foods.

Re: Genetically Modified Organisms (GMO):
There is no US law that requires that GMO food
be labeled as such.
So, we cannot know which foods are or are not
GMO.
Buyer Beware.

Avoid also, Soda and Diet Soda, Corn Syrup,
High Fructose Corn Syrup, Agave, (which
contains more fructose than even high fructose
corn syrup).

For more about "sugar as a toxin," google
Robert Lustig, MD, from the department of
pediatrics at the University of California, San
Francisco, who has proven that **the rise of
chronic disease is linked to higher sugar
consumption.**

These studies are about "added" sugar" only.
The sugar that is in foods naturally, like an
apple, is fine.

Avoid Packaged foods, and any product that
lists in the ingredients "Natural Flavor,"
"Fragrance," Food Colorings and Dyes.

Natural Flavors

"Natural flavors" are very different from what consumers might expect.
That is because they can contain both artificial and synthetic chemicals (often used as processing aids).

The label "natural flavors" could be a mask for unhealthy and toxic ingredients.

Not all "natural flavors" are inherently dangerous for human consumption.
But, the label "natural flavors" has come to indicate that they are not that natural.

The term "natural flavors" is often used to camouflage potentially dangerous ingredients.
The term is very loosely regulated by the FDA.
The FDA defines "natural favor" under CFR - Code of Federal Regulations Title 21
as "whose significant function in food is flavoring rather than nutritional."

A company or manufacturer is free to label any flavor as natural, as long as it is derived from a natural substance even though it is chemically modified.

The FDA does not require companies to list what the natural flavors are, so the consumer has no way of knowing.

Personally, I avoid anything that has the words "natural flavors" in the ingredient list.

Stevia

Use Organic Stevia instead of sugar or other sweeteners.

Do not use Truvia. It contains erythritol (an unhealthy sugar alcohol) and "natural flavors."

Needless to say, do not use any of the following: Aspartame, Acesulfame potassium, Alitame, Cyclamate, Dulcin, Equal, Glucin, Kaltame, Mogrosides, Neotame, NutraSweet, Nutrinova,

Phenylalanine, Saccharin, Splenda, Sorbitol, Sucralose, Twinsweet, Sweet 'N Low, or Xylitol All have serious permanent and short term harmful effects on your health They cause too many very serious illness and disorders to list. https://draxe.com/artificial-sweeteners/

Canned food

BPA is a toxic chemical that causes hormone imbalances and wide variety of health issues ranging from hypertension, aggression, obesity, to cancer and heart disease. There are no regulation or safety standards regarding the amount of BPA in canned foods.
https://www.womenshealthmag.com/health/the-dangers-of-eating-canned-foods

Oils

Best oil is Organic, Virgin, Cold Pressed, Unrefined Coconut Oil, for cooking, frying, and baking.

> "Coconut oil supports thyroid function, normalizes insulin and leptin sensitivity, boosts metabolism and

provides excellent and readily available fuel for your body in lieu of carbohydrates." Dr Mercola articles - https://tinyurl.com/y9x2zpnu

It is said that saturated fats are not healthy. But that is a myth.

Saturated fat got a bad rap more than 60 years ago by the American Heart Association who coupled saturated fat with trans-fatty acids and proclaimed coconut oil as "pure poison."

The American Heart Association took on the cause against saturated fats and has never updated its stance with the latest research and facts.

Trans-fatty acids are the worst type of dietary fat. It is a by-product of a process called hydrogenation that is used to turn healthy oils into solids and to prevent them from becoming rancid. Trans fats have no known health benefits and there is no safe level of consumption. They are outlawed in the

US. Coconut oil does not contain any trans-fat.

Organic Olive Oil is okay for salads but not for cooking – it oxidizes and becomes carcinogenic.

Avocado oil, and Almond Oil are healthy oils.

Never, ever, use Canola oil, Vegetable oil, Soybean Oil, Cottonseed oil as a food.

Packaged Foods

Avoid packaged foods, and foods labeled "sugar-free" or "gluten-free."

I avoid any package that has a list of more than three ingredients.
Eat only foods that do not need such a label, like vegetables, nuts, fish etc.

Read the ingredients.
If you don't understand them or know what they are – Don't Eat Them!

Meat or chicken should be USDA Organic, Free Range, Grass Fed and Grass Finished, No Antibiotics, No Hormones, No rBST, no CAFO (Concentrated Animal Feeding Operations) meats.

Drink lots of Water but . . .

Drink lots of water, but only filtered or bottled water, preferably without fluoride. NY State mandates Fluoride in all their drinking water. Fluoride is a neurotoxin and a hormone disrupter. (Read a little further for more on fluoride in drinking water.)

Beware, also, of bottled water that has chemicals added.
For example, Kirkland Water adds the following: potassium bicarbonate, sodium bicarbonate, calcium citrate, and magnesium oxide.

These are not healthy or appropriate additives to be imposed on every person drinking their water.

Also, I am wary of water that sits in plastic bottles. This tells me that soaking in plastic means some of that plastic dissolves into the water.
It is admitted that "plastic bottles made from PET (Polyethylene Terephthalate)
will leach very small amounts of antimony which is a heavy metal.

Food-safe plastic containers can contain a chemical called Bisphenol A, or BPA. BPA is an endocrine disruptor, meaning it interferes with your normal hormone function and especially disrupts estrogen.
BPA leeches from its plastic source and enters food and water.
There are bottles that are BPA free but a BPA-free water bottle could be just as toxic as your old BPA-rich Nalgene."
"Items that are free of BPA often contain other chemicals that behave in much the same way – leaching into foods and drinks. After being

absorbed by the body, the chemicals mimic the hormone estrogen, increasing the risk of cancer, diabetes, obesity, and reproductive problems." (https://www.mensjournal.com/health-fitness/why-bpa-free-plastic-isnt-necessarily-safe-20140611/ https://www.cnn.com/2016/02/01/health/bpa-free-alternatives-may-not-be-safe/index.html)

More about Fluoride

The public has been misinformed to believe that fluoride builds bones and strong teeth.

In reality, fluoride is highly toxic.
It damages your immune system, causes teeth to get blackened (fluorosis) and bones to be brittle.
If that is not bad enough, it also causes cancer.

Fluoride in your drinking water does absolutely nothing to strengthen your teeth or bones.

On top of that, every fluoridated toothpaste has, in tiny print, the following warning on the box and on the tube:
"Keep out of reach of children under six years of age."

Yet, even though it is toxic to children (and adults), one must wonder why toothpaste is flavored like candy, rather than with something that prevents it from being eaten like candy.

The labels on the tube warn us that "If you accidentally swallow more than what is used for brushing, then seek professional help or "contact a poison control center immediately."

The mouth is very absorptive and so more likely to be poisoned by what we put in our mouths than by what is put on our skin.

The American Dental Association seal of approval cautions:
"Don't Swallow — Use only a pea-sized amount for children under six,"
and
"Children under 6 should be supervised while brushing with any toothpaste to prevent swallowing."
The word "poison" is not used, even though it is a poison.

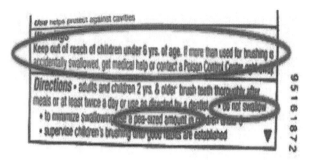

Fluoridated Water Causes Underactive Thyroid

"Studies have shown that iodine deficiency may be caused by extra ingestion of fluoride and is related to hypothyroidism."
https://tinyurl.com/ycvs7vq4

A recent study:
A 2012 study led by Stephen Peckham of the University of Kent in Canterbury, England found that in locales where tap water fluoride levels exceeded 0.3 milligrams per liter, the risk for having an underactive thyroid rose by 30 percent.

Peckhams' team also found that hypothyroidism rates were nearly double in urbanized regions that had fluoridated tap water, compared with regions that did not.

Also, avoid Juices, Soda, Diet Soda, Artificial Sweeteners including Equal, Splenda, Sweet & Low, Saccharin – they are highly toxic and Carcinogenic.

Do Eat Organic fruits and vegetables.

Do Not Cook in Aluminum pots or pans, or non-Stick pots or pans. Aluminum gets into the food and causes conditions such as Alzheimer's.

Check all your:
Cleaning Products and soaps and shampoos – read the ingredients:

Avoid products with SLS (Sodium Lauryl Sulfate), Titanium Dioxide, Triclosan (in Antibacterial liquid soaps), Fragrance, FD&C

colorings, Household chemicals, Toothpaste, Hair Dyes, nail polish, skin creams, etc.

Cell Phones – Don't wear a cell phone on

your body.
Avoid Bluetooth
headsets.
Use the speaker phone
whenever possible.

Put the phone down on the table, not in your hand.

Keep your cell phone at least 6 inches from your body.

Do not sleep with a cell phone next to you.
Keep your phone at least 3 feet away from you, especially while charging it or when you are not using it.

> **Everything we think, everything we feel, every emotion, and everything we put on or into our bodies, affects our health.**

Reaction of Others

I have experienced that people often get really disturbed by my not eating.

At an event like a wedding, a luncheon, or a gathering of people, when I first began eating this way, some would keep asking "Can you eat this? … And what about this?"

The truth is that after having given up those foods that are not healthy for me, I have zero desire for them.

It is not challenging at all to go to places
where there is cake, or ice cream, or meat,
or anything that I no longer partake of.

I am so grateful to I feel great without those
foods that there is no temptation
whatsoever to take even a taste.

I go to events, and meals with others for the
company, not for the food.

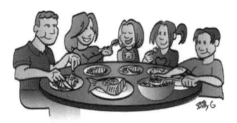

Chana Klein

How I Learned that Cancer LOVES Sugar

Before the PET Scan at Beth Israel Hospital Radiology Center, I asked what they were injecting into my body.

The hospital person told me it is a radioactive sugar, called fluorodeoxyglucose.

He explained that I would have to wait an hour for the scan after being injected so that

the injected liquid will reach my cancer
cells.

He described how the sugar in the injected
substance makes a bee line for the cancer
cells, highlighting the location of the cancer.

Anywhere the sugar accumulates (in the
cancerous tumors) shows up like a light
bulb on the scan.

That is how they know where the cancer is.
The sugar goes directly to the cancerous
tumors.

Chana Klein

In other words, Cancer loves sugar.

Sugar goes directly to,
and feeds the cancer.
Sugar makes the cancer
grow.

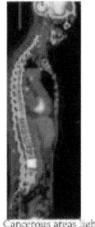

http://usaided2013.net/page/2

Cancerous areas light up

I later found out that
cancer cells consume
15-times more glucose
than normal cells do.
That is what makes the
radioactive glucose so effective in finding
the cancer.[1]

Light FROM the Darkness of Illness
& Physical Disability

[1] In 1926 the Nobel prize winner Otto Warburg wrote that glucose represents one of the main energy sources of cancer. and some tumors when deprived of glucose can die. And if they do not die at least they will continue to grow at a much slower rate and will be weaker and susceptible to other treatments such as chemo.
The Metabolism of Tumors in the Body by Otto Warburg, Franz Wind, and Erwin Negelein
Warburg, O, Biochem.Z 1923 cxlii 317. Warburg, O , Poener, K and Negelein, E. Biochem Z 1924, clii, 309, etc.

That is what I heard.

So, of course, the first food I gave up was

processed sugar.

Because I had no appetite to begin with, it

was not difficult for me to give up any food.

When I returned to eating, I always kept the

image in my mind of cancer growing from,

and feeding on, sugar.

With that in mind, and the memory of how horribly ill the cancer caused me to be, it is not difficult to steer clear of sugar.

No Resistance

I continued to go to Pilates sessions and to do the techniques I have learned in my Eden Energy Medicine trainings, NET training, Guided Imagery training, Chinese Medicine training, etc.

I did not "fight" my illness.
I just went on living.
Unable to keep my head up or to speak

without passing out, I did only what I was
able to do.

Sometimes, all I could do was to lie in bed
and watch a DVD.

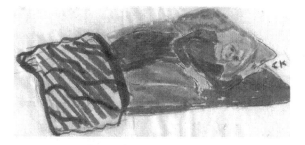

After a few months passed, I had watched
all the documentary DVD's in the Teaneck
library.

Then I began watching movies.

I did not resist my cancer in any way.

I was even resolved to it taking my life.

But my not resisting, it seems to me, made
the cancer not resist me.

Not resisting it, allowed the cancer to relax
and to flow out of my body.

The cancer did not
become stuck, unlike the
tiger in this picture that is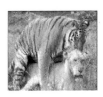
holding on more tightly to the lion, the
more the lion resists.

Fighting something causes it to hold onto us
more tightly.

I never again went for another test.

At this writing, it's nine years since my

diagnosis and I feel amazing, full of energy,

clarity, and full of life.

My not resisting,
it seems to me,
made the cancer
not resist me.

Chana Klein

The Lesson

What we resist persists.
What we are okay with becomes okay.
What we focus on grows.

I focus on my life,
on what I am doing
today,
on what I am really
feeling now,
on what I have,
on whom I love,
and I am okay.

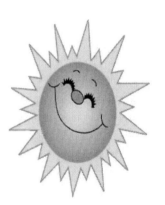

The More I Resist . . .

The more I resist the rejection of another, the more rejected I get.

The more I try to make you love me, the sooner will your rejection come.

The more I resist feelings of depression, the deeper the depression goes.

The more I try to fall asleep, the more alert and awake I become.

Chana Klein

The more I try to look pretty, the less attractive I appear.

The more I try to be an intuitive, the less my intuition serves me.

The more I try to convince you that I am right, the sooner will you find me wrong.

The more I try to appear smart, the more errors I make.

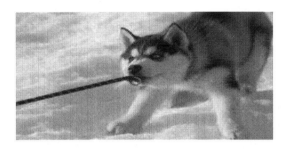

The more I try to get my children to tell me
things, the less they share with me.

The more I try to do everything myself,
the less I get done.

The more I resist and fight an illness,
the more ill I become with it.

The more I try to avoid stress, the more stress chases me.

The more I resist, the more my problems persist.

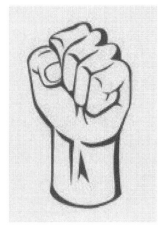

Finding Victory in Retreat

Finding victory over illness by not resisting, began, perhaps, as long ago as Avraham in the Book of Genesis.

Avraham Avinu (Abraham, our Forefather) found victory in retreat, victory in NOT resisting.

The story as told by Rav Soloveitchik: "Abraham was told to withdraw, and to defeat himself by giving Yitzchak away."

Chana Klein

(This is known as "The Akeida" – "The Binding of Isaac".)

In other words, when Avraham was told to sacrifice Yitzchak (Isaac), his favorite son, even though it must have seemed like an outrageous command, he did not resist God's command.

Instead, Avraham got Yitzchak ready by tying him up on an altar and preparing him as a sacrifice for God.

Avraham was preparing to be defeated in
this most important area of life without any
resistance.

He was just following what he heard God
tell him to do.

Because Avraham did not resist, (and also
because God does not want human
sacrifice,) God sent an angel to stop
Avraham from performing the sacrifice and

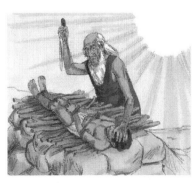 Yitzchak
was
returned to
him.

Chana Klein

He (Avraham) listened to God.

God accepted the God-fearing intentions of

Avraham and his preparations for the

sacrifice of Yitzchak.

But God did not take Yitzchak.

God returned him to Avraham.

(Genesis 22:17)

Avraham enjoyed another 75 years with

Yitzchak, until Avraham passed to the next

world at age 175. (Genesis 25;7)

In this way, Avraham found victory in

retreat.

Confrontation and other Essays by
Rabbi Joseph B. Soloveitchik, p. 40,
Maggid Books (2015)

(This Learning was inspired by
Rabbi Menachem Meier, Shlita.)

Avraham's victory came to him because he
was willing to be defeated.

He was ready and willing to lose his most
precious possession.

He did not resist, or fight God's command.
Avraham simply did what God told him to
do.

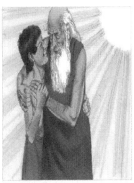

And the result was that Avraham achieved victory in having his son restored to him.

http://www.freebibleimages.org

Avraham needed this test in order to become Avraham, the Father of the Jewish Nation, which is the meaning of his name.

He did not resist and that was part of his greatness.

The Cure is Created Before the Illness

There is ALWAYS hope.
All things are possible.

The Torah talks about the *Refuah* (the healing) being created before the *Makkah* (the sickness.)

That means the remedy was created before the illness was created.

Chana Klein

The Torah is telling us that there is already
a remedy for each malady before it even
occurs.
We just need to access it.

In other words, the healing remedy was
created before the disease was created.

In more modern terms, if nature created the
disease, then nature also created the cure.

The healing is there for us before we even
search for it.

We need to search though, and to be open
and proactive when we find it.

Light FROM the Darkness of Illness & Physical Disability

(See my story: The Power in the Search)

Once again, we can embrace our illness experience.
We can use our cancer, or any illness, as an opportunity to find our Light FROM the Darkness.

Cancer can make us better than we were before its occurrence, through the life lessons it teaches us once we survive it.

Cancer can be life changing making us better or making us worse.

It is our choice.

The hoops we go through in being ill and in getting better, as painful as they are, build our character

They force us
to grow if we
choose to see it
that way.

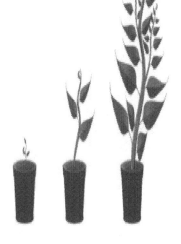

Light FROM the Darkness of Illness & Physical Disability

And once the storm is over, you won't remember how you made it through, how you managed to survive.

You won't even be sure whether the storm is really over.

But one thing is certain. When you come out of the storm, you won't be the same person who walked in. That's what this storm's all about.

Haruki Marakami

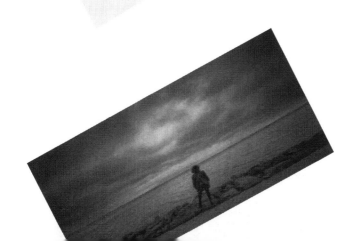

Chana Klein

FROM WHERE IS
OUR HELP?

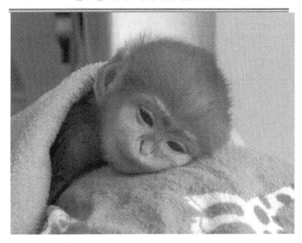

From Where Will My Help Come?

A diagnosis, an awful diagnosis.

Many of us have been through one or two or more upsetting diagnoses, either for ourselves, for our child, for our spouse, for our friend, or for someone close.

It's devastating.

In my practice, I often must address the emotional effects of just hearing the diagnosis before dealing with the actual illness.

348

Chana Klein

We experience shock, fear, anger, grief, and
other complicated reactions.

Our heads flood with confusion, with:

What do I do now?
Will I be able to function?
Will this make me ugly?
Why is this happening to me? Etc.

We fill with fear of what is, of what will be,
fears of things that usually do not happen,
but still affect our health negatively.

In the dark, we remain awake, in the middle

of the night,

imagining.

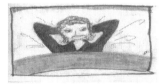

In the shower, we are ruminating.

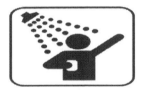

Between sips of a hot drink, and bites of

food, we obsess.

Chana Klein

We have become preoccupied and suffer

low energy because of hearing the

diagnosis.

We each, in our own way, ask:

From where will my help come?

King David asked that very question in

Psalm (Tehillim)121

> A song for ascents.
> I shall raise my eyes to the
> mountains, from where will my help
> come?
> My help is from the Lord, the Maker
> of heaven and earth.
> He will not allow your foot to falter;
> Your Guardian will not slumber.
> Behold the Guardian of Israel will
> neither slumber nor sleep.

> The Lord is your Guardian; the Lord
> is your shade; By your right hand.
> By day, the sun will not harm you,
> nor will the moon at night.
> The Lord will protect you from all
> evil; He will guard your soul.
> The Lord will guard your going out and
> your coming, in from now and to
> eternity.

This psalm is asking what so many of us ask

when we are ill:

Where am I going to get my help?

King David provides the answer.

The psalmist raises his eyes to the

mountains and concludes

"My help comes from God."

Chana Klein

According to the Rabbis of the Talmud

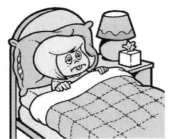

(Nedarim 40a), help comes from God's personalhttp://cliparts.copresence (the Shechinah) which is above the head of a sick person. (Rashi Gen 47:31)

This is so important for each of us to know.

God's Presence When We Are Sick

Knowing that the Shechina (God's presence) is above the head of the sick person means that when I am in pain, or going through withdrawal from a medication, or burning with fever, or weak from anemia, or whatever is ailing me, I keep in mind that according to Chazal (Our Jewish Sages), God is with me, as He personally stays with the sick.

This makes me feel better.

Avraham

We see this first with Avraham. God Himself personally visits Avraham when he is recovering from his circumcision.

Then God even sends three angels to him with different messages.

God is certainly paying attention to Avraham while he is ill.

But is it just for a great one like Avraham? Or is it for each of us when we are ill that we get the actual presence of the Almighty.

God's Presence

According to The Torah, the *Shechina* (God's presence) hovers over the head of each person who is ill.

The Gemara (Talmud) tells us that because God's presence is with the sick person, a visitor is required to cover oneself with a prayer shawl when visiting. (Nedarim 40a)

The reason for that requirement is because entering the room of a sick person means you are entering God's presence.

And more:

The visitor is not even allowed to sit on the bed, or on a stool, or a chair in the room of the *choleh* (sick person) because God's presence rests there.

> The Gemara notes that **this is also taught** in a *baraita*: **One who enters to visit a sick person may neither sit on the bed nor sit on a bench or on a chair** that is higher than the bed upon which the sick person is lying. **Rather, he** deferentially **wraps himself** in his garment **and sits on the ground, because the Divine Presence is resting above the bed of the sick person, as it is stated: "The Lord will support him upon the bed of suffering,"** and it is inappropriate for one to sit above the place where the Divine Presence rests.   Nedarim 40a

How does that affect an ill person in bed to know that God's presence is at the head of his bed?

To know that God is truly with him/her! Wow!

The invalid, we read in the same passage, has no vitality at all. It is only the divine presence that gives him life.

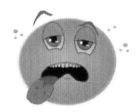

S

Chana Klein

God Cares for Us When We Are Sick

Our Torah tells us in so many places that God is with the *choleh (sick person)*.

The Talmud further shows us how God personally cares for each one of us who is ill:

> Rabbi Yoḥanan said: Anyone who requests that his needs be met in the Aramaic language, the ministering angels do not attend to him to bring his prayer before God, as the ministering angels are not familiar with the Aramaic language, but only with the sacred tongue, Hebrew, exclusively.
>
> (Shabbat 12b)

> The Gemara responds: A sick person is different. He does not need the angels to bring his prayer before God because the Divine Presence *(already)* is with him.

359

This tells us that the prayer of a sick person

goes straight to God.

Sometimes we don't feel that or realize it.

But for me, it helps to know.

And another:

> **For Rav Anan said** in **Rav's name: From
> where is it derived that the Divine
> Presence cares for** and aids **the sick
> person?**
> **As it is stated: "God will support him on
> the bed of illness"** (Psalms 41:4) (Shabbat
> 12b)

God Feeds Us When We Are ill

Beyond that, Chazal teach that God is the One who feeds the ill during illness.

I wonder if that is why I didn't need food when I had cancer!

> Rava said in the name of Raven: **From where** is it derived **that the Holy One, Blessed be He, feeds the sick person** during his illness?
> **As it is stated: "God will sustain him on the bed of illness."** (ibid)

ss

From Where Will Come My Help?

It is clear, at least to me, that our help when we are ill (and also when we are well) is from the Almighty.

We need to be aware of that, and to not hesitate to ask Him for help.

In Psalms (Tehillim) 147:3, God is called *HaRofei* - The Healer.

362

It is really God who does the healing.

The Gates of Tears

The sages say that ever since the destruction of the Second Holy Temple, the "gates of prayer" are closed.

On the subject of prayer, **Rabbi Elazar also said: Since the day the Temple was destroyed the gates of prayer were locked** and prayer is not accepted as it once was, **as it is said** in lamentation of the Temple's destruction: **"Though I plead and call out, He shuts out my prayer"** (Lamentations 3:8). Yet, **despite** the fact **that the gates of prayer were locked** with the destruction of the Temple, **the gates of tears were not locked,** and one who cries before God may rest assured that his prayers will be answered, **as it is stated: "Hear my prayer, Lord, and give ear to my pleading, keep not**

silence at my tears" (Psalms 39:13). Since this prayer is a request that God should pay heed to the tears of one who is praying, he is certain that at least the gates of tears are not locked.   Brachos 32b

Rabbi Eliyahu Dessler explains that with prayer that emanates from deep within the heart to the point that the supplicant is moved to tears, one can achieve results. This gate is never closed.
Michtav MeEliyahu IV p 262

The "gates of tears" are always open.

> *"Every gate has been locked shut except for the gates of tears."*
> *Bava Metzia* 59a

While God closed the "gates of prayer," in His eternal mercy, he kept open the "gates of tears."

This means that when we are suffering so much that we have tears, we can go to Him with our tears and know that our plea is reaching Him.

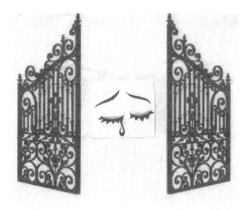

We can know that we are heard.

What this means to us is that when we cry, it is more beneficial to direct our cries to God, rather than to self-pity.

Light FROM the Darkness of Illness
& Physical Disability

Have you noticed personally that sincere tears
directed to the Almighty create change for you?

The gates of tears remaining open means that
any time we are in pain, in sorrow, in fear, we
can cry out to Hashem with our tears and He
hears us.

It means that when we cry, God notices.

Often healing seems impossible, as if there are
no cures and no solutions.
But we ask for help, and suddenly and
miraculously, help appears.
We get better!

Take Advantage

I know terrible things happen. They have certainly happened to me. Read my first book *Light FROM the Darkness: A Different Perspective on Difficult Times,* if you doubt that.

But even with that, I know for sure that every time I cry out, God hears me and cares.

Light FROM the Darkness of Illness & Physical Disability

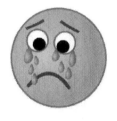 When I cry out with true tears, I find that things change.

Miracles happen.

The God I know wants good for us, even though people have free will to hurt each other.

God especially watches over the sick.

He leaves a path for our tears to go straight to Heaven, when we cry to Him.

A caveat: Be careful to not complain as the Jews did in the wilderness.

Also, please don't cry from self-pity.

Chana Klein

Rather, cry to God with your plea.

Enlist Him with a sincere cry requesting

what you need.

God loves you.

He cares.

He is there for you.

Know that and take advantage.

With gratitude to Rabbi Daniel Fridman, Shlita of Teaneck Jewish Center for introducing me, during his Rambam shiur, to the concept that God stays at the head of the bed with the sick person, and for providing many of the sources quoted on that.

369

LESSONS FROM MY NEAR-DEATH EXPERIENCE

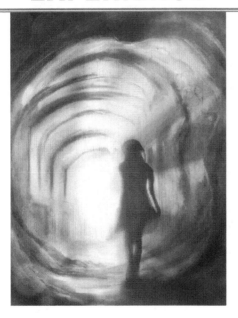

Chana Klein

Does It Matter?

"So, I did a small thing. It didn't hurt anyone. No one will ever know."

I wonder how many of us have thought
such thoughts.
Is it true that it will never matter, whatever
it is, or was?

I had borrowed a set of tape cassettes from a
Jewish organization in the 1980's.
I listened to each tape more than once.

Then, I forgot to return them.

Light FROM the Darkness of Illness
& Physical Disability

Cleaning out my attic more than twenty
years later, I saw the set of tapes lying in the
disorganization that had been up there.
I didn't know what to do with them.

These cassette tapes are sort of useless now,
I told myself.
Most people, are listening to CD's and
iPods, not cassette tapes.

I felt ashamed that I had not returned the
cassettes.
I felt I would be judged if I told someone
that I had failed to return something,
judged by people, that is.

Chana Klein

I did have a passing thought that I might be
judged by Heaven.
But the important thing to me at that
moment was saving face in the here and
now, with people.

In reality, it may not have seemed to be
such a great sin.
Perhaps it was what we call a *chait*, missing
the mark, a mistake.

But as my soul sees it now, the price was
too great to ignore it.

Light FROM the Darkness of Illness & Physical Disability

In August 2009, I was deathly ill. I had been so ill that I literally passed to the other side.

When I got there, I was given a very enthusiastic welcome by my brother, Michael, A"H, who had died in 1992. He seemed to be waiting for me and seemed to be exhilarated to see me.

I, later, wondered how my brother knew that I was coming. I also wondered why he was alone there, the only one greeting me.

I realized that I had expected a crowd of people to be there when my time was up.

Chana Klein

I don't know who exactly I was expecting,
other than my brother.
But, just the same, it was not what I
expected.

As Michael stood in front of tall beautiful
green bushes, he lured me to join him.

I suddenly felt a vortex-like-tunnel pulling
me back to the healing table where my
physical body rested in a fetal position,
unable to feel itself.

My (ex) husband was working on my
lifeless body, using the EEM healing

techniques we had spent years being trained in.

But the formidable force of my brother's welcome, again, pulled me back to the very bright place where he was animatedly standing, luring me.

There were no peepholes in the bushes to see what lay on the other side of them.

My brother, who had been very ill when he died, now looked terrific, happy, and healthy.

Chana Klein

And then again, Whoosh! I felt the vortex-
tunnel grabbing me back to the healing
table and to my (ex-) husband.

And then I was again pulled back with
Michael.
I was drawn back and forth, with no sense
of time.

I awoke (at about 4 am) to see my (ex) -
husband in his tallis (prayer shawl), praying
at my side.

It was clear then, that it was almost
morning and that I was going to be alive in
this world, at least for another day.

Light FROM the Darkness of Illness & Physical Disability

Perhaps, as a result of my encounter with that world, my vision is clearer than it had been before.

That clarity has remained with me as I write this book.

It's as if issues, things, actions, have sharper, clearer edges.

There is a defined contrast between what is good and what is not, and a clear picture of results and consequences of each action.

What about the cassettes?

I was still in a quandary about exactly how to handle that.

In the next world, I had a vision of myself in
how I dealt with the cassette issue.
I was paying dearly in the next world for
my mistake.

I soon heard a speaker tell a story of how,
more than 20 years ago, he had taken
something that was not his from an
institution.

He shared that his rabbi suggested that he
send them a donation to correct his act.
Hearing that story was a personal message
for me.

I followed through with a meaningful contribution to the institution, worth more than the unreturned cassettes, to correct my mistake, along with a copy of this story for the rabbi to read.

Until this experience, I had gone through my life journey, unaware of how Heaven does justice.

This taught me that each deed is so much more meaningful and important than I could have imagined.

I am so much more aware, now, of how significant my intention is in every little thing I do.

I can no longer just be carefree or careless in my actions and decisions.

I now see the sparks and the energy that each thing we do generates.

Every little thing we do is recorded. All our actions are important. Everything counts.

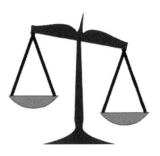

There is more about how we are judged that
is revealed in the next story, The Only Way.

The Only Way

How Are We Judged by Heaven Where It Really Counts?

Does God judge us the way people do?
How are we judged in Heaven,
where it really counts?

Was it a Punishment?

Arnie Greenstein, A"H passed to the
next world during the week that we

read the Torah portion known as Parashat
Shemini.

> The sons of Aaron, Nadav and Avihu, each
> took his firepan, they put fire in them and
> placed incense upon it; and they brought
> before Hashem, an alien fire, that He had
> not commanded them.
> A fire came forth from before Hashem and
> consumed them, and they died before
> Hashem. (Leviticus 10:1-2)

Was this a punishment?

They did what they were *not* commanded

and died as a result of what they did.

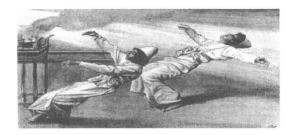

But it may not be so simple.

God, here, is called by the name that

represents his attribute of Mercy, rather

than Judgement.

That makes me wonder if being consumed

is an   from the death of Nadav and Avihu by James Tissot

actual punishment?

The passage does not say.

It says that they were consumed.

It does not say they were killed.

It says they "died before God."

Consuming involves making something a

part of you.

Is that what God was doing?

To explain the death of Aron's two sons, Moshe repeats God's words to him, "I will be sanctified through those who are nearest Me. Thus, I will be honored before the entire people; And Aron was silent." (Leviticus 10:3)

Those words, also, do not communicate judgment, but rather closeness.

Arnie

Arnie was a member of the Carlebach Shul in Teaneck, NJ.

Light FROM the Darkness of Illness
& Physical Disability

He had the appearance of being homeless,
although he may not have been.
Arnie had been suffering from failing
health.

Despite the pain he always seemed to be
experiencing and his apparent difficulty
breathing, he biked to a Torah class every
day, struggling to travel miles to get there.

Arnie was loved by many members of the
Carlebach Shul minyan.

But the way he dressed, or didn't, often
having an odor, his appearance, and what
goes with that, might lead others to feeling

superior to Arnie, as if they are better than, holier than, more righteous than he is.

Despite the way he was treated by the loving people of the Carlebach shul, people still judged him, avoided him, and felt superior.

It was no accident, but rather a life lesson for each of us, in how we judge another person, that Arnie went to the next world during the week of Parshat Shemini.

What About Us?

Something happens to us and often, we think it is a punishment for something we have done.

How does what Nadav and Avihu did, and the consequences of their actions, apply to us?

Does the story help to explain whether God judges us the way people do?

Chana Klein

How are we judged in Heaven, where it really counts?

My Story

From 2007 through 2009, I had been very ill. I eventually lost my vital signs and spent a brief time in the next world.

Understandings, that became ingrained in my soul, rendered me unable to forget all that I learned at that time.

Nothing in this world has looked the same as it did before that experience.

Light FROM the Darkness of Illness
& Physical Disability

I saw, there, that reward and punishment
are not what I had thought they would be.

While I saw, on the one hand, that every
little thing we do counts more than we
could ever realize, I also discovered that
God is much more understanding of our
misdeeds than I could have ever imagined.

I saw my brother, Michael, there.
He was the one to greet me.
He and I had had it very tough when we
were children.

Chana Klein

He ended up doing what I saw as terrible
things to cope with the harsh treatment we
received.

Yet, Michael ended up looking so well up
there.
He seemed in such a high place.
I saw that he was clearly good.
He earned it, perhaps with the Teshuva
(repentance) he did before he passed to the
next world, and perhaps even more, with all
the suffering that he had endured during
his life.

What was very clear to me was that God
understood the why of what Michael had

done, the what, and "the who" of who my

brother really was.

The Only Way We Could Be

God saw Michael do what he did, and it looked to me that He did not afflict him because of it.

I realized that the things Michael did, the choices he made, may have been the only things that he could have done and the only way that he could be.

God sees us and understands our actions more than we understand ourselves.

Chana Klein

God sees and understands our mistakes.

At the same time, He sees our greatness and
what we could be.
God also sees what we cannot be.

How many of us are the only way that we
could be?

Perhaps that is the way we are supposed to
be.

Light FROM the Darkness of Illness & Physical Disability

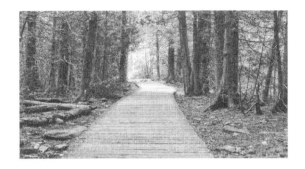

"Everything I thought was a
mistake,
Every street I thought was the
wrong street,
Turned out to have been the only
way to get there."
    Rabbi Shlomo Carlebach

For me also, there is so much in my

background that could make me feel shame.

Chana Klein

There are people I know who have what we
call *Yichus* (heritage, lineage, relatives) of
great people who did important things.
I have none.

While Michael and I were growing up, I
searched for one relative to look up to as
someone from whom to seek wisdom.

The search was in vain.
In the communities in which I am involved,
I could easily feel
shame of where I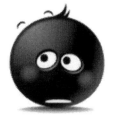
came from and how I
grew up.

Yet, I wonder if the way it was had really been the only way to get to where I am now.

If I had not seen what I saw, if I had not been where I had been, would I have been able to merit the guidance of my Creator as I did and still do?

Would I have been able to even recognize it as such?

What is really good?
And what is really bad?
How can we know for
sure?

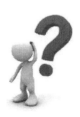

Chana Klein

How can I look at the actions of another and
appoint myself as judge?

How could I have looked at the actions of
my own brother and think I know better, or
that I have done better?

How do I know that was not the only way
for him to get to where he was going?

How do I know that where I have been, is
not the only way for me to get to where I
am supposed to be going?

Even the smallest shift in perspective
can bring about the greatest healing.
Joshua Kel, The Quantum Prayer

Changing Perspective

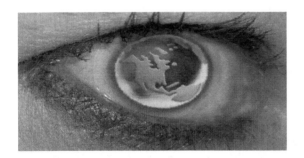

When we visit a mourner we seek to comfort him or her.

Chana Klein

In Hebrew this is called being *"Menacheim Avel."* (Consoling a Mourner)

But the real meaning of *"Menacheim"* we learn in Genesis 6:6, when God *reconsiders* (*VayiNacheim* Hashem) having created man. *Nacheim* means to change one's perspective. (as taught by Rabbi Yosef Adler, Shlita)

So, when we are being *Menacheim Avel* to someone, our visit with them is hopefully changing their perspective.

The verses on the death of Nadav and Avihu in our Torah, plus my own

experience when floating in and out of the
next world, have changed my perspective.
It has removed any judgment I may have of
how any one chooses to live.

Perhaps as Rabbi Carlebach stated, that is
the only way that person can go.
"Nachamu, Nachamu, Ami," ("Be
comforted, be comforted, My people,") the
prophet Isaiah tells us. (Isaiah 40:1)

Perhaps the comfort for me, the change in
perspective today, is to know that my road
was right for me, to know that Arnie's road
was right for him, to know that some of
those "streets" that seemed to be so wrong

and even cruel, were really the way that the Almighty wanted each of us to go.

"Nachamu, Nachamu," the comfort is to know that it was okay.
To know that I chose the way that I was supposed to.
"Nachamu Nachamu," God is my comfort."

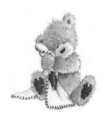

Death Wish

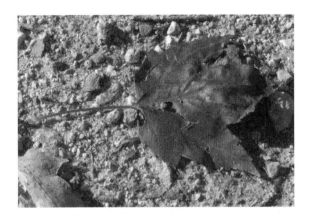

I used to wish I were dead.
I used to pray to be dead.

I imagined that death would be like going to
sleep;
Only, my life would be over.
I would never have to wake up again;

never again have to experience the physical
pain,
or the perennial shock at how others treat me.
I would never again have to experience the hate
and shunning from others.

I just wanted it all to be over.

I had worked so hard.

It was not in my nature to give up while I was
alive.
Only death would allow that.
I felt I had done enough already.
I knew I had tried my best in each situation.

"No more pain! Please, God. I want to be dead!"
I never stopped talking to God.

Light FROM the Darkness of Illness & Physical Disability

I cried to Him, yelled at Him, thanked Him.
Whatever I was feeling, I stayed in relationship
with the Almighty.

But that did not stop me from praying that He
take me away from the savagery that I
experience in this world.

"Wish I was dead!" became my mantra.
I often said it out loud without even realizing.

It was the early 1980's.

I was the Spanish teacher in a small New Jersey
town.

My classroom was on a cart.
I wheeled the cart to different classrooms.

Chana Klein

The teacher of the class would go on a break
while I taught Spanish, using puppets, games,
drama, and everything I could create for my 6th
to 8th grade students.

The school provided me with a closet behind the
auditorium stage to keep all those teaching
materials.
The closet floor measured 5'7" long x 4' wide.

How do I know?
Did I measure it?

No! I would put a pillow on the floor and

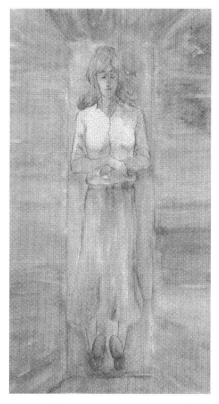

lie down
for part of
my lunch
break.

The closet
was
about an
inch
longer
than the
height of
my body.

I fit perfectly.

Even had some space for my stuff.

During my lunch break, I would lay my head on the pillow and meditate on the most comforting image I could think of:

> "This is my coffin. It's all over. I don't have to live through another day or another hour, for I am now dead, here, in my coffin."

That image lulled me to a 15-minute relaxation and sleep to renew my energy for the rest of the day.

But these thoughts were nothing new.

Light FROM the Darkness of Illness & Physical Disability

As far back as I can remember, I had always held onto the idea in the back of my mind that I would have an "out."
I would take my life.

As a matter of fact, I planned it.
Part of that plan was to work on clearing my garage to make room for my car.

Then, I strategized, that I would close the garage door, run the gas, and in some way, end my life.
Just like they did in the movies.

My brother, Michael (A"H) used to ask me on the phone, "How is your garage?"

Chana Klein

Michael knew I was clearing it and why. We both understood that the clearer the garage was, the worse my life felt and the closer I was to ending it.

When the
garage was
cleared
enough to
fit the car
in it, I
would

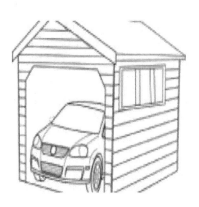

have a way to do it.

We both understood that this dialogue was about my plan.

Ending my life was my relieving thought.

It meant the torture could end.

Then, in the 1980's, I heard a rabbi comment

in class that a person who kills himself can't

have a place in the afterworld.

It had nothing to do with The Torah portion

we were learning.

He just mentioned it in passing.

I couldn't believe it.

I never heard that before.

Now, what recourse did I have?

Chana Klein

I didn't comment other than to clarify what
he said.

I had to make sure I'd heard him right.

I didn't want to do something to give
myself more agony.

Of course, he never told us that Jewish law
considers a person who does this as
mentally ill.

Also, he did not share that the act is not
considered unforgiveable under certain
circumstances.

> Rabbi Yechiel Epstein, in his classic work the
> *Arukh HaShulchan* (Yoreh De'ah 345:5)
> states, "This is the general principle in
> connection with suicide: we find any excuse
> we can and say he acted thus because he

> was in terror or great pain, or his mind was
> unbalanced, or he imagined it was right to
> do what he did because he feared that if he
> lived he would commit a crime...It is
> extremely unlikely that a person would
> commit such an act of folly unless his mind
> were disturbed."
> (http://tinyurl.com/y8rg6h8t)

But at the time, I imagine that I was not supposed to hear all that.

Now, after that learning, ending my life was no longer an option for me.

Still, when I heard of someone's early death, I envied that person.

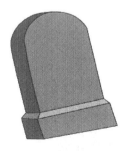

The Lesson of My Life (or Death)

And decades after, I had the lesson of my life . . .

Or was it the lesson of my death?

Aggressive cancer (from which I eventually healed myself naturally) made me very anemic and feverish for a full three years before I was diagnosed.

I remember my call to Rabbi Weinberg telling him that I don't feel any life-energy within me. I was feeling loss of life force, or death, encroaching my body.

Light FROM the Darkness of Illness
& Physical Disability

Even though I became weaker and weaker, I
chose not to go to a hospital.

I felt that one dose of chemo would likely
kill me.
I was too weak for anything that was the
slightest bit invasive.

On that day, (that I called Rabbi Weinberg,)
I knew I was not going to make it through
the night.
I just knew.

Laying my head in my lap while at the
computer, unable to keep my head up, I still

worked at completing the Ethics Rules
document for the Professional Association
of ADHD Coaches (PAAC).

I got it done.

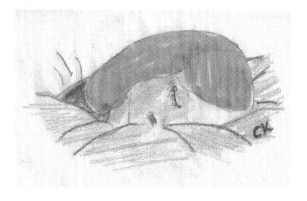

I emailed it to three of the board members
with a note saying that I don't think I am
going to make it through the night.

Of course, having ADHD, none of them
opened it for another week.

I also returned the PayPal payments of any
clients who had prepaid.
I added a note that I don't think I will make
it.
I left out the part that said, "through the
night."
I was steering away from the "drama
queen" within me.

A few days before this, I had been rushed to
Beth Israel Hospital where I was given a
transfusion of several units of blood.

But the weakness this night went even deeper.
I was going in and out of consciousness. I could not use my voice without passing out.

Only for my youngest son, did I work so hard to muster up the energy to say a few words on the phone.

Loving him as I do, I did not want him coming over and pushing me to go to the hospital.

"I can't let him hear how sick I am."

Then, I felt myself going through a huge

vortex.

I was no longer in my body.

I could see my body lying on my healing

table in a fetal position, as if I were floating

above it.

I did not feel anything.

Yet, I had full consciousness.

I viewed the crown of my husband's head.

I saw him wearing his tallis looking at the

prayer book in his hands.

I saw my brother Michael in the next world

luring me to come past those very alive,

gorgeous, green bushes that he was

standing in front of.

And images of so much of my life were

flashing before me.

I saw clearly what mattered.
I saw what I should have fixed.
I saw what did not matter . . .
Everything became so clear.

But what became the clearest was that death

does not mean it's over.

I had left my sick body.

But I never really went to sleep as I had
imagined I would when I die.

Death did not mean a loss of being
conscious of my life or of the people in it.

It only meant to me that there is nothing
more I can do now to change anything.

Death meant that I was now stuck with
what I had done during my days here in
this world.

I saw that while I had remained here, I
could have fixed it.
I could have fixed almost anything.

But in death, there are no changes that I
could make.

What I had believed that I was seeking in
death did not exist.

Death is not really the end.
It is only the end of opportunity to fix it and
to make it better.

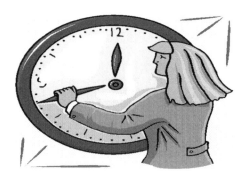

Our Patriarchs and Matriarchs Asking God for Death

Was I a bad person for wishing to be dead?

Is it a great sin to ask God to take my life?

Was my wish to be dead so unusual?

Many prophets of God had times when they stated their own wishes to be dead.

I find this mind blowing, as well as comforting and freeing.

Let's look at our matriarchs and prophets and see their words in the simple text of the Tanach (Bible):

Rivka

"Rebecca said to Isaac, 'I am disgusted with living because of these daughters of Heth; if Jacob takes a wife from among the daughters of this land, from Hittite daughters, like these, my life will not be worth living."
(Genesis 27:46)

Is that a death wish or what???

She is saying that if it is not her way then she wants to die.

Rachel

And there is Rachel:
And when Rachel saw that she did not bear children to Yakov, Rachel had jealousy toward her sister and said to Yakov,

"Give me children, or else I die."

 (Genesis 30:1)

Again, no mistake about Rachel wishing to die.

Chana Klein

Moshe Rabbeinu (Moses)

Even the greatest prophet of all time, the man who spoke face to face with God, our Moshe Rabbeinu, had times when he asked God to kill him:

> "I, alone, cannot carry this entire
> nation, for it is too heavy for me.
> If this is the way You deal with me,
> then, **kill me now,** if I have found favor
> in Your eyes, so that I not see my
> misfortune."
> (Bamidbar/Numbers 11:14-15)

And it's not limited to The Torah.

425

Our prophets:

Elijah

He (Elijah) came to a broom bush and sat down under it and prayed that he might die.

> "Enough!" he cried. "Now, Oh Lord, take my life, for I am no better than my fathers."
>
> (I Kings 19:4)

Jonah

We read Jonah's request for death just before the afternoon prayer of

Yom Kippur. That is, before the holiest
moment on the Jewish calendar.
(The Epilogue of this book says more on
Johah's death wish.)

Jonah "begged" God for death!
Didn't I do the same?
Maybe not at his
level.
But to me it was
begging.

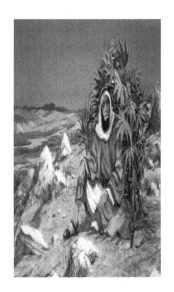

And what was the
problem for Jonah
that made him want
to die?

A plant???

How many trivial things make us feel we

want to die?

How many big things?

Life is not easy.

It's not supposed to be.

We're supposed to reach, to strive for better,

to search, to ask for, to question.

We're supposed to grow through our

terrible troubles, to grow our soul.

Jeremiah

And then, I must tell you, this next one horrified me when I read the full text, which you can do on your own.

OMG Jeremiah is so poignant
and sooo real!

This is what he writes:

> Accursed be the day that I was born, the day
> that my mother bore me.
> Let the day not be blessed!
> (Jeremiah 20:14)

And Jeremiah is one of our major prophets,

whose words we read in the Haftorah on

holidays of Tisha B'av, Rosh Hashanah, and several specific Sabbaths.

If it was okay for Jeremiah, then it is likely okay that you or I have had such thoughts and prayers.

The Rabbis of the Talmud

Even the rabbis who are quoted in the Talmud ask if it is better we should not have been born.

The question itself suggests that the rabbis thought about not being alive.

Chana Klein

For two-and-a-half years, the School

of Shammai and the School

of Hillel debated.

> These said, "It is better for man not to
> have been created than to have been
> created"; and these said, "It is better for
> man to have been created than not to
> have been created."
> (Talmud, Eruvin 13b)

The Death Experience

For me, in my death experience, I could
see more of this world than I could

when I was here in this world.

The clarity became so much greater.

But I could not do anything about any of it.

Light FROM the Darkness of Illness
& Physical Disability

I could not change anything.

I could not influence my children, or help
my friend, or write my thoughts.
I could not do anything other than know
about it.

The thing I wanted to do most during my
life was to change and grow.
That could not happen once I was no longer
alive.

Every situation that is difficult in my life is
still an opportunity to make a change, to fix
something, to grow.

Once my soul leaves this world, I will know, of that I am sure . . .

I will know what is happening and what has happened.

But I will no longer have the opportunity to fix anything.

Getting Ready

I found that it is easier to get ready to die than to get ready to live.

Getting ready to die involves saying good bye to my things, to people, putting things

away, getting them in order, deciding to
whom I want to give my belongings, etc.

But getting ready to live is much more
complicated and difficult.

Getting ready to live means facing choices,
life changing choices.

It means terminating some relationships
that are not healthy for me, and it means
having the courage to begin new
relationships.

It means also having the courage to be
alone.

Chana Klein

It means continuing to work on myself in overcoming what stops me.

It means taking steps forward, when sometimes I would rather hide my head in my pillow.
It means speaking up for myself.

It means confronting rejection and failure, as well as encountering hard work and success.

It means being present for whatever shows up in my life, and being okay with it all.

Getting ready to live is a beginning.

Light FROM the Darkness of Illness & Physical Disability

Getting ready to die, is so much easier.

Once I saw that I was no longer immanently dying, the great challenge was getting ready to live.

That meant the challenge of cleaning up my life.

Returning to this world with the gift of the clarity and the insight I received in the next world, presented the opportunity to fix everything that I saw in the visions.

Chana Klein

I so appreciate that I can be here to fix my life, and hopefully to be a positive influence on the lives of others.

At this time, in what is becoming a long life for me, I have no wish to be dead.

I am grateful that I can see more clearly and that I can work at fixing my life, at helping my family, my friends, my clients, and adding to the fixing of the world.

Each of us can still do that, if, and when, we choose to, during our lifetime.

Light FROM the Darkness of Illness
& Physical Disability

Facing my suffering has unlocked my
strength and even more.
It has unleashed such joy inside of me,
the joy that shines from deep down, every
day,
the joy that turns a destructive Hurricane
Sandy into an opportunity to meet more
people and to be there for them, the joy that
sees opportunity in everything and that
increases the recognition that my greatest
challenges are the key to my strength, and
to my understanding.

Chana Klein

"There is no
way to get to
the next world
by escaping this
world.
Only by
mastering it."

(Rabbi Simcha
Weinberg,
Shlita)

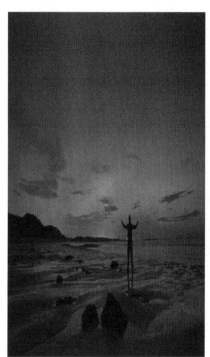

That is the
Light FROM the Darkness

EPILOGUE

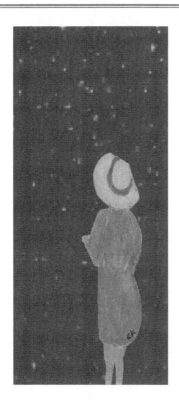

Chana Klein

I wrote this book to help you to understand yourself, why you may be ill, why you remain ill, and how to really heal.

I was set up in this world to become a very ill person, given the infanthood, childhood, teenage years, and the young adulthood that I suffered.

Read my first book, *Light FROM the Darkness: A Different Perspective on Difficult Times,* for more on that.

But all that horror has turned into a Light FROM the Darkness for me, as it has added to my ability to help others.

Light FROM the Darkness of Illness & Physical Disability

It has privileged me to become a part of the healing journey of each person with whom I work.

All the torment with which I lived helps me to understand the pain of another, not only as a professional, but as a person who has been through the same, and often, even worse, and who has come out whole, healthy, and happy, with the ability to help others to do the same.

That is the Light FROM the Darkness.

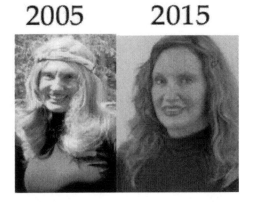

Chana Klein

Today in my more mature years, I am healthier than I have ever been, and I keep getting better.

I was recently given a photo that was taken of me in 2005.

Compare it to the photo of me two years ago (2015), and then to the photo on the

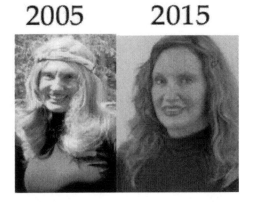

book cover taken the year I am writing this book (2017).

The first two photos are included in my presentation entitled: *The Face as the Subconscious: How to Read the Wrinkles and How to Clear Them*, which I gave to an International Group of Eden Energy Practitioners.

In my practice, I use the face as a way to see what is happening in the body, and the emotions.

The state of our health, emotional and physical, shows on the face.

Chana Klein

Our face shows what is happening, or has
happened, inside the body, and the mind.

My presentation to the group showed how,
as we face our darkness, our health and
mind improve and with that, wrinkles often
clear, as they did with me.
Wrinkles do not have to be permanent.

I had many more wrinkles in 2005 when my
health was failing.
As I healed on the inside, so too, did my
wrinkles disappear.

Illness is stuck energy.
Stuck emotions create that stuck energy.

Stuck energy is what creates wrinkles on the face, showing as lines, mountains and valleys.

Facing my darkness has relieved the stuck energy that created wrinkles.

In general, each wrinkle has a different emotional source, stemming from a different body part or organ.

For example, the condition of the heart shows on the tip of the nose, while the condition of the pancreas shows on the upper bridge of the nose.

Chana Klein

The chin reveals inflammation of the
kidneys and bladder caused by fear.
Exhausted adrenals appear on the lower eye
lid which drops under stress.

The under eye reveals more about the
kidneys.

I could go on explaining what the face
shows us.

But I think you have the idea, now, of the
importance of the face in reading the body
and emotions.

Light FROM the Darkness of Illness & Physical Disability

I share this to show that wrinkles and skin quality reflect our state of health and that facing our darkness clears our health issues and our wrinkles.

The clearing of wrinkles is an indication that the body, the mind, and the spirit are healing.

The healing I have experienced is a result of what I have shared in this book about Dark Cures Dark.

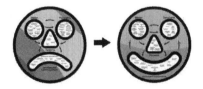

One more lesson I wish to share:

A REAL CONVERSATION WITH THE ALMIGHTY

We learn a lesson about getting Light FROM Darkness by understanding what a Jew reads in synagogue, on the holiest day of the year.

Not only the holiest day, but before the holiest moment!

449

That is, the moments before the Neilah prayer of Yom Kippur.

The Neilah Prayer is recited as the sun is going down.
It is the time of the "closing of the gates of prayer" as Yom Kippur is ending.

During Neilah, the heavenly judgment that was inscribed on Rosh Hashanah is being sealed.

The shul fills with stirring pleas to have our prayers accepted by God, before the holy day of Yom Kippur ends.

Chana Klein

Why is The Book of Jonah read as the prelude to this prayer?

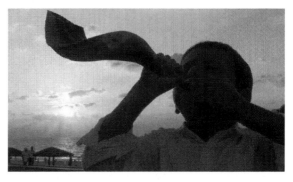

Why do we read Jonah at this most holy of moments?

The Story

Jonah admonishes the city of Nineveh, warning them to repent before the city will be destroyed in 40 days.

The people of Nineveh believe Jonah, turn
away from their wickedness, and God
shows them mercy.

But Jonah, now, becomes angry and bitter
because God did not destroy the Ninevites
who were Israel's enemy!

On the holiest moment of the year, we read
about *anger* and *bitterness* of our main
character, Jonah.
Why this reading?

Then, when Jonah sits to rest, God provides
a vine to give him shade.

The next day, God sends a worm to eat the
vine.

Jonah is now sitting in the hot sun
complaining and wanting to die.
Jonah actually cries to God that he wants to
die.

He asks God to kill him.

> "And now, O Lord, take now my soul from
> me, for my death is better than my life."
> (Jonah 4:3)

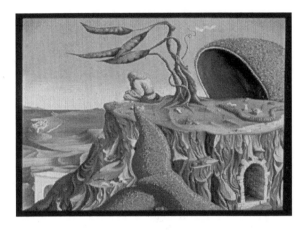

And then Jonah *begs to die*:

> "Now it came to pass when the sun shone, that God appointed a stifling east wind, and the sun beat on Jonah's head, and he fainted, and he _begged to die,_ and he said, 'My death is better than my life.'"   (Jonah 4:8)

Chana Klein

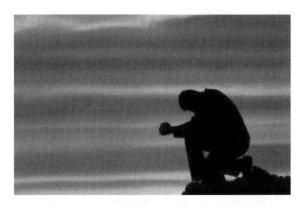

And we read this as a prelude to the holiest moment of the year!

On the day that we are trying to be sealed in the Book of Life, we are reading about the main character who is begging to die.

Jonah is facing his darkness.
He is being real with himself and with God.

Light FROM the Darkness of Illness
& Physical Disability

Over a little thing like a plant, he says he
wants to die.

How many of us feel such darkness over
what appears to another to be a little thing?

That is how Jonah feels and that is what he
expresses to the Almighty.

Does the Almighty punish Jonah for such a
terrible request?
It does not seem that way.

We are reading the story of a character in
the Tanach stating the darkest feelings
anyone could feel.

Chana Klein

We read this model of a real conversation
with the Almighty!
Jonah expresses anger, bitterness, death
wishes, the ugliest of feelings.

Yet, we read this as a prelude to the holiest
moment of the year.

What does this show us?
I believe it shows us that God wants us to
share with Him our real feelings, our
darkness, even what we see as our ugliness.

God is showing us real teshuva
(repentance), real healing, by having us
express the real us, the real Jonah.

God wants us to be real.

Dark cures dark.
Teshuva in the book of Jonah means being
real.

It guides us to be honest and authentic with
God and with ourselves.

And Jonah is the model of that.

Chana Klein

Why else would God have us read a story in
which the main character is full of anger
and begs for death?

I believe that God is showing the way for
each of us, in the importance of being
authentic with what we really feel.

I see this especially as a message for those
who are trying so hard to be "good" or
"nice" and in the process, discounting their
true feelings.

When hurt or disturbed by someone or
something, they often say, "that's okay."

Light FROM the Darkness of Illness & Physical Disability

For those who are being so nice while holding their real feelings in . . .

For those who believe that a negative thought is not allowed under God . . .

For those who think that all thoughts must be filled with loving goodness . . .

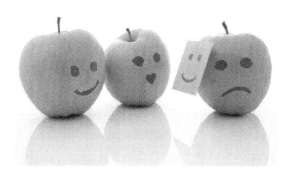

Chana Klein

Is that what God wants?

Are we supposed to be forever positive and
sweet in our prayer and conversation with
the Almighty?

If so, why is the model on Yom Kippur,
Jonah?

Why, of all the readings that could be
chosen as a prelude to Neilah, was Jonah
chosen?

I have found that God wants us to be
authentic.

At the same time, I have also found that being authentic is what creates healing.

How can we be authentic unless we feel what we really feel, rather than what we think we should feel?

What a freedom!
What a relief!
That it's okay to feel whatever I feel and if I am real with myself, I will heal.
Does it get any better?

This is having a real conversation with the Almighty, a real relationship.

462

Chana Klein

Being real.

That is what God wants from us.

That is what the Universe requires in order

to keep us healthy and clear of stuck

emotions, clear of toxic feelings,

clear of environmental toxicity, and getting

healthier and healthier.

Be who you are and not who you, or others,

think you should be.

Be real, not sweet, unless that is how you

really feel.

God loves the Real You!

Of course, we must always treat every

person with great respect.

I am referring here only to the *real*

conversations between you and the

Almighty.

I bless each of you to know what you really

want, to find it, and to be who you really

are.

ABOUT CHANA KLEIN

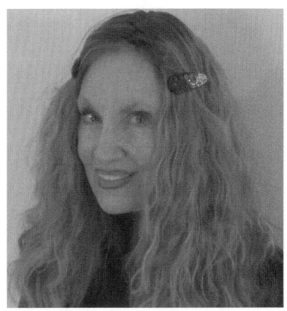

Chana Klein, MSEd, PCC, EEM-AP, MCAC, ACG, PACG, CCUG, EFT, NET, AGI, SSS®, CBT-I

Light FROM the Darkness of Illness & Physical Disability

During Chana's bout with cancer, she had a near-death experience.

In *Light FROM the Darkness of Illness & Physical Disability*, Chana shares the lessons gleaned in the afterworld that changed her life and her perspective.

She came back from there with increased clarity, which she uses in her life and in her work.

Chana's early world of emotional and physical trauma granted Chana an indomitable spirit that never gives up.

Chana Klein

She learned, through an inordinate amount of disabilities and illnesses, to work and work until she gets where she wants to be. That is how Chana works with each client.

Having completed endless trainings and certifications in Healing and Coaching, she has learned to be a healing detective in finding the source of each problem and how to fix it.

In doing the detective work to find what will work for each client, Chana does not give up until each one is well, or free of whatever caused him/her to seek her help.

Light FROM the Darkness of Illness & Physical Disability

Chana, with God's help, healed her own Stage IV Ovarian Cancer nine years ago (as of this writing).

In addition, she healed her Reflex Sympathetic Dystrophy (RSD), her Candida, her numerous bone issues, hormonal issues, heart issues, blood sugar problems, anxiety, panic, insomnia, addiction, countless health issues, and paralyzing learning disabilities of ADHD, Dyslexia, Dyscalculia, et al.

Chana's trainings and experience have turned her into an almost magician, able to heal maladies like Cancer, RSD, Multiple

Chana Klein

Sclerosis, Parkinson's, Mental Illness, Emotional Problems, Depression, Panic, Trauma, Tourette's, and just about every illness that walks in her door.

Her clients report that one session of the work that Chana does has been more effective than years of therapy in getting the results they seek.

Chana's trainings have given her the basis to develop her own techniques for working with those diagnosed with Autism Spectrum, Schizophrenia, OCD, and a myriad of mental disabilities.

Light FROM the Darkness of Illness & Physical Disability

Through the practice of the techniques and concepts in this book, Chana has been able to reach her own truth and has guided her clients to reaching theirs.

Chana has been studying the writings of The Torah, spending between 3 to 6 hours/day in Torah classes since 1980.

Much of her insight into healing has been affirmed for her in her Torah studies, and she shares many of The Torah sources of her insights in this book.

Light FROM the Darkness of Illness & Physical Disability: What Makes Us Ill, What Keeps Us

Chana Klein

Ill & How to Heal explains Illness and Healing, as Chana has mastered, through decades of learning and experience with clients, as well as personal experience in overcoming her own illnesses and disabilities, and those of her many clients.

For Chana's stories and insights into Illness & Mental Disability, read her next book:

Light FROM the Darkness of Invisible Disability &Disorder: True Stories of Understanding & Recovery from Learning Disability, ADHD, Autism, & Other Brain/Body Wirings
to be published shortly.

Chana would love to hear from you:

chana@lightfromthedarkness.com

Chana's websites:

https://lightfromthedarkness.com

https://theadhdcoach.com

https://thespectrumcoach.com

Your review of this book on Amazon

would be very appreciated.

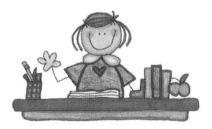

Notes:

Notes:

Chana Klein

Notes:

27686593R00261

Made in the USA
Columbia, SC
30 September 2018